"Dr. Geyman advocates for single-payer health care with his usual wit, reason, and immaculate documentation. This time he fortifies his points with personal stories from across the country, describing the wreckage left by the Affordable Care Act. Putting human faces on ObamaCare brings the argument home poignantly. The people telling their stories of our failed health care system could be our friends, our families, and us. The unhappy consequences of ObamaCare touch us all."

—Samuel Metz, M.D., adjunct associate professor of anesthesiology,
Oregon Health and Science University, Portland, OR

"This book has heartbreaking stories of U. S. citizens who face medical and financial catastrophes due to our dysfunctional healthcare system which now includes the ACA.

We need to listen to these stories to feel the true impact of how the profit-based medical industry is harming our society. A major paradigm change to single-payer is discussed as an equitable and viable solution.

—Ray Drasga, M.D., long-time community-based oncologist and leader
toward universal health care in his own specialty organization,
the American Society of Clinical Oncology.

"Many liberal Democrats supported ObamaCare as a step toward a universal single-payer public health insurance system. As Dr. John Geyman's book makes clear, ObamaCare was instead a leap into the arms of a rapacious private insurance industry that hiked premiums, denied care, cancelled policies, narrowed networks, jacked deductibles, drove doctors to burnout, fueled the rise in medical costs, raided the public treasury, bloated the bureaucracy and corporate profits, privatized Medicare and Medicaid, decreased the quality of care, and left 30 million Americans uninsured. Next time, can we learn from this debacle? Read this book. Then just say no to the private health insurance industry and those who would play their deadly game."

—Russell Mokhiber, Single Payer Action

D0958932

"Although many had high hopes for ObamaCare, as John Geyman shows us the human faces, we realize that reform fell too short for too many. He shows us not only those human faces but also the pained face of health care justice. He provides us with an understanding of what is wrong with our system, and then describes options for the future. He encourages us all to participate in the reform dialogue so that we can finally get this right. The Human Face of ObamaCare is a great place to start."

—Don McCanne, M.D., family physician, senior health policy fellow and past president of Physicians for a National Health Program (PNHP).

"In his latest book John Geyman takes stock, honestly and objectively, of the state of American health care five years into the implementation of ObamaCare. He examines the law's effects on our healthcare system, on the healing professions, and on individual Americans and makes a persuasive case the ObamaCare is unsustainable. He presents three possible scenarios for future reforms.

After reading this comprehensive and persuasive critique, I am more convinced than ever that an improved and expanded "Medicare for All" system is not only the best for the vast majority of Americans but is the only reasonable option for those of us who believe health care should be focused on the prevention and treatment of illness rather than wealth-extraction from patients.

The only question now is how much longer the public will tolerate the accelerating corruption of our healthcare system Geyman documents and the charade that masquerades in Washington as a real debate about health care policy.

This book is a must read for any American who has been or will be exposed to the American healthcare system. That would be all of us."

—Philip Caper, M.D., internist with long experience in health policy since the 1970s, and past chairman of the National Council on Health Planning and Development

"Dr. Geyman has done it again: another up-to-the-minute report on the current state of our ailing health care system. This time, he includes a report card on the first five years of the Affordable Care Act, where it has succeeded and failed, and his forecast of what may come next. Like everything else he has written, his research is thorough and remarkably current. Where others rehash yesterday's statistics and arguments, Geyman's books are like breaking news. In this book he makes the facts personal: faces and cases of recurring failures in our privately-insured and profit-driven system to meet the medical costs of our people when they're sick. The system is still broken in 2015, Geyman explains, and it is breaking us. Finally, unlike so many critics of ObamaCare, Geyman shows us a rational and practical way out."

—Rick Flinders, M.D., family physician and inpatient program director,
Santa Rosa Family Medicine Residency, Sutter Santa Rosa
Regional Hospital, Santa Rosa, CA

"Dr. John Geyman gives us a clear summary of failed incremental reform attempts over many decades. The Affordable Care Act, AKA ObamaCare, is the latest example, and Geyman highlights its many shortcomings, including perverse incentives, rising costs, narrow choices, and still-incomplete coverage. He concludes with a cogent, compelling argument for a single-payer national healthcare system: the approach that's worked everywhere else in the world."

—Richard Deyo, M.D., Kaiser Permanente Professor of Evidence-Based
Family Medicine, Oregon Health and Science University,
Portland, and author of Watch Your Back!

"An insightful critique of ObamaCare and an impassioned plea for a single-payer system, enlivened by stories of real people poorly served by the Affordable Care Act. An invaluable contribution to the discussion of how to make health care in America better and more affordable for everyone."

—Kenneth Ludmerer, M.D., professor of medicine and the history
of medicine at Washington University in St. Louis, and past
president of the American Association for
the History of Medicine

Also By John Geyman, M.D.

The Modern Family Doctor and Changing Medical Practice

Family Practice: Foundation of Changing Health Care

Family Practice: An International Perspective in Developed Countries (Co-Editor)

Evidence-Based Clinical Practice: Concepts and Approaches (Co-Editor)

Textbook of Rural Medicine (Co-Editor)

Health Care in America: Can Our Ailing System Be Healed?

*The Corporate Transformation of Health Care:
Can the Public Interest Still Be Served?*

Falling Through the Safety Net: Americans Without Health Insurance

Shredding the Social Contract: The Privatization of Medicare

The Corrosion of Medicine: Can the Profession Reclaim its Moral Legacy?

*Do Not Resuscitate: Why the Health Insurance Industry is Dying,
and How We Must Replace It*

*Hijacked: The Road to Single Payer in the Aftermath of
Stolen Health Care Reform*

*Breaking Point: How the Primary Care Crisis
Endangers the Lives of Americans*

The Cancer Generation: Baby Boomers Facing a Perfect Storm
Second Edition

*Health Care Wars
How Market Ideology and Corporate Power Are Killing Americans*

*Souls on a Walk:
An Enduring Love Story Unbroken by Alzheimer's*

*How ObamaCare is Unsustainable:
Why We Need a Single-Payer Solution for All Americans*

The Human Face of ObamaCare

Promises vs. Reality
and
What Comes Next

John Geyman, M.D.

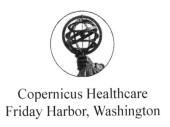

Copernicus Healthcare
Friday Harbor, Washington

The Human Face of ObamaCare
Promises vs. Reality and What Comes Next

John Geyman, M.D.

Copernicus Healthcare
Friday Harbor, WA

First Edition
Copyright ©2016 by John Geyman, M.D. All rights reserved

Book design, cover and illustrations by W. Bruce Conway
Author photo by Anne Sheridan

softcover: ISBN 978-1-938218-02-6

Library of Congress Control Number: 2015953361

Copernicus Healthcare
34 Oak Hill Drive
Friday Harbor, WA 98250

www.copernicus-healthcare.org

Dedication

To the countless millions of Americans struggling under the cost and access burdens of our increasingly dysfunctional health care system. May they and future generations finally have a system that works for all of us, with service for all, not profits for the few, its dedicated goal.

The Human Face of ObamaCare:
Promises vs. Reality and What Comes Next

Table of Contents

PART ONE
A Myriad of Problems and Experiences

PART TWO
System Trends under the Affordable Care Act

PART THREE

What Comes Next? Three Alternatives With Different Futures

Tables and Figures

ACKNOWLEDGMENTS

As with my previous books, I am indebted to many for making this book possible. First, I have appreciated the constructive comments by these colleagues who reviewed selected chapters:

- Howard Brody, M.D., Ph.D., Director of the Institute for Medical Humanities, University of Texas Medical Branch, Galveston

- Philip Caper, M.D., internist with long experience in national health policy work dating back to the early 1970s, past chairman of the National Council on Health Planning and Development, and founding member of the National Academy of Social Insurance

- Richard Deyo, M.D., MPH, Kaiser Permanente professor of evidence-based family medicine, Oregon Health and Science University, Portland

- Rick Flinders, M.D., inpatient program director, Santa Rosa Family Medicine Residency, Sutter Santa Rosa Regional Hospital, Santa Rosa, CA

- Larry Green, M.D., Epperson-Zorn chair for innovation in family medicine, University of Colorado, Denver

- David Himmelstein, M.D., general internist and professor of public health at City University of New York and co-founder of Physicians for a National Health Program

- Don McCanne, M.D., family physician, senior health policy fellow and past president of Physicians for a National Health Program (PNHP)

- David McClanahan, clinical associate professor of surgery emeritus, University of Washington School of Medicine, and coordinator of the Western Washington Chapter of Physicians for a National Health Program, Seattle, WA

- Samuel Metz, M.D., adjunct associate professor of anesthesiology, Oregon Health & Science University, Portland, OR

- Charles North, M.D., MS, professor of family and community medicine, University of New Mexico and former chief medical officer, Indian Health Service

- Steffie Woolhandler, M.D., general internist and professor of public health at City University of New York and co-founder of Physicians for a National Health Program

I am also grateful for the helpful suggestions of colleagues who looked over the entire manuscript, including:

- Mark Almberg, communications director for Physicians for a National Health Program, Chicago, IL

- Don Berwick, M.D., president emeritus and senior fellow, Institute for Healthcare Improvement and former administrator, Centers for Medicare and Medicaid Services

- Ben Day, executive director, Healthcare-NOW!, health care analyst and activist toward universal health care

- Ray Drasga, M.D., long-time community-based oncologist and leader toward universal health care in his own specialty organization, the American Society of Clinical Oncology

- David Gimlett, M.D., family physician and former medical director of Inter Island Medical Center, Friday Harbor, WA

- Kenneth Ludmerer, M.D., professor of medicine and history at Washington University in St. Louis, and past president of the American Association for the History of Medicine

- Ted Marmor, Ph.D., professor emeritus of public policy and political science, Yale School of Management, and author of *The Politics of Medicare* and *Fads, Fallacies and Foolishness in Medical Care Management and Policy*

- Russell Mokhiber, executive director of Single-Payer Action, Washington, D.C.

- David Satcher, M.D., Ph.D., director of Satcher Health Leadership Institute at Louis W Sullivan National Center for Primary Care, Morehouse School of Medicine, Atlanta, GA and former U.S. Surgeon General

- Margie Schaps, executive director, Health and Medicine Policy Research Group, Chicago, IL

- Wendell Potter, former CIGNA executive, senior fellow on health care at the Center for Media and Democracy, and author of *Deadly Spin: An Insurance Company Insider Speaks Out On How Corporate PR Is Killing Health Care and Deceiving Americans*, and *ObamaCare: What's In It For Me? What Everyone Needs to Know About the Affordable Care Act*

Thanks are also due to many investigative journalists, health professionals and others for their probing reports on our dysfunctional health care system. The work of many organizations has been helpful in putting together an evidence-based picture of what is actually happening in U. S. health care, especially reports from the Centers for Medicare and Medicaid Services (CMS), the Center for National Health Program Studies, the Commonwealth Fund, the Congressional Budget Office (CBO), the General Accounting Office (GAO), the Kaiser Family Foundation, the Organization for Economic Cooperation and Development (OECD), Public Citizen's Health Research Group, the U. S. Census Bureau, and the World Health Organization (WHO).

As with previous books, Bruce Conway, my colleague at Copernicus Healthcare, has done a great job with this project from start to finish, including book design of the interior and cover, typesetting, and conversion to ebook format. Carolyn Acheson of Edmonds, Washington, has created a reader-friendly index.

Most of all, I am indebted to my new wife, Emily, for her suggestions and encouragement through the entire process; she has read every bit of the manuscript over its various iterations, bringing her eagle-eye to editing and proofing, and also helping with promotion of the book.

PREFACE

Now that the Affordable Care Act (ACA) has been upheld by the U.S. Supreme Court as the law of the land, it is the target of an intense partisan debate during this 2016 election cycle. Confusion, disinformation, and misleading rhetoric dominate the airwaves as politicians and their corporate backers offer up wildly different approaches to our health care problems and solutions.

After six years with the ACA, there is a large base of experience to draw upon to assess, on the basis of evidence, what has worked and not worked. So it is time to reassess its impacts on the problems it was intended to address—reduced access to health care, uncontrolled costs, increasing unaffordability, and unacceptable quality of care for our population.

Despite promises of the Obama administration before the law was passed that we can keep our insurance if we like it, stay with our same doctors, and save money at the same time, many millions of Americans have too often found these assurances to be empty. Having insurance "coverage" for many does not translate into having access to affordable necessary care. Instead, the largely for-profit "system" continues on, profiting and sometimes profiteering from expanded markets subsidized by us, the taxpayers. The original title of the ACA as the Patient Protection and Affordable Care Act (PPACA) has become a misnomer, not surprisingly little used today.

Too we are often bombarded by abstract numbers and statistics that neglect what they mean to ordinary Americans. This book takes a different approach, starting with stories of patients and their families, thereby putting a human face on the large body of experience and evidence about the effects of the ACA since its passage in 2010. Far from isolated anecdotes, these are common stories that best illustrate national trends and problems in our increasingly dysfunctional market-based system.

The book is organized in three parts: Part One presents some 50 patient and family stories that represent problems confronted by implementation of the ACA since 2010. These are real people and their families drawn from press reports. Part Two looks at five major problems of the entire system, as we consider to what extent the ACA has addressed them, and find that we are far from the health care reform that we need. Part Three deals with where we are now, in the middle of an election year, faced with three main alternatives about where to go next: (1) stick with the ACA or try to improve it; (2) repeal and replace it with a Republican "plan"; or (3) move to single-payer system of national health insurance. You will notice that many of the chapters start with a heading, "The Promise", "The Premise," or "The Myth." These denote either the promises made by the Obama administration about the ACA or the premises underlying it, which typically and ironically are based on earlier conservative ideas put forward by conservative organizations, such as the Heritage Foundation.

The stakes are too high to get health care wrong in this country. Our incremental reform attempts over many years have been compromised by the money and political power of corporate stakeholders that perpetuate many of our problems. We need objective evidence to combat the rhetoric and claims of the medical-industrial complex and direct our attention to the real needs of patients and their families. It is my hope that this book will help in this process.

—John Geyman, M.D.
Friday Harbor, WA
January 2016

PART ONE

A Myriad of Problems and Experiences

CHAPTER 1

I HAD INSURANCE,
BUT IT WAS CANCELLED

From the beginning, we were assured by the Obama administration that we could keep our health insurance if we liked it. The Affordable Care Act would not get in the way of our existing coverage. It would just add new opportunities to get new coverage if uninsured, or give us a chance to improve our coverage through a more competitive marketplace.

But many Americans have found this to be untrue, as these examples illustrate.

> *Edie Littlefield Sundby, who lives in San Diego, California, is a seven-year survivor of stage 4 gallbladder cancer, which has a five-year survival rate of less than 2 percent after diagnosis. Insured by a United Healthcare PPO (preferred provider organization) since 2007, her doctors and treatment teams have been in California (Moores Cancer Center at the University of California San Diego and Stanford University's Cancer Institute) and in Texas (MD Anderson Cancer Center in Houston). "My affordable, life-saving policy was cancelled effective December 31, 2013. My choice then was to get coverage through my state's ACA exchange, Covered California, and lose access to my cancer doctors, or to pay much more for insurance outside of the exchange, with quotes averaging 40 to 50 percent higher. After four weeks of researching plans on the exchange and talking to counselors, insurers, and providers, my in-*

surance broker and I are as confused as ever. Although I have had great care and solid insurance through United Healthcare for more than six years, that coverage is gone. United Healthcare has paid $1.2 million to keep me alive since 2007. I have been fortunate to have continuity of care by my excellent doctors over this time, and now am forced to lose that continuity at much higher cost. If I go with the exchange plan, I must choose between Stanford, which has kept me alive, and UCSD, which has provided emergency and local treatment support, including my primary care doctors. What happened to the promises with the ACA that you can keep your insurance and your doctor? For a cancer patient, medical coverage is a matter of life and death."[1]

Kristine Stewart Hass, a 49-year old freelance writer and editor and married mother of five, had her health insurance plan cancelled because of not meeting the ACA's requirements. She had been paying nearly $300 a month for it with a $5,000 deductible. She was able to get a bronze plan on the federal exchange, but now pays $581 a month for family coverage with a deductible of $12,000. Although she qualifies for a subsidy, that will only help with about $300 a month, and this new coverage is barely affordable and leaves her with having to deal with a huge deductible.[2]

Lance Taylor, a 64-year old retired commercial real estate broker in Victorville, California, had a plan covering himself and his daughter cancelled, again because it didn't meet the ACA's requirements. He had been paying $431 a month with an annual deductible of $6,000. He found a replacement policy, but it costs $731 a month, covers unwanted maternity and newborn care coverage, and he doesn't qualify for a subsidy.[3]

Dave Osterfield, a 61-year-old retiree, who now trades stocks, was happy with his insurance plan covering himself and his wife until it was cancelled. The reason given was that it didn't meet the ACA's requirements. He had been paying $400 a month with a $10,000 deductible. He balked at having to pay $1,000 a month for a replacement policy with a family deductible of more than $12,000.[4]

Fraser Ratzlaff, a 33-year old in Seattle working for a Christian non-profit providing for orphaned and destitute children, had his "bare-bones" catastrophic insurance coverage cancelled after the ACA took effect. He had been paying $100 a month for that coverage. Last year, he obtained new coverage that included all the free services that the ACA requires, but his premium doubled, and even then he was paying for benefits he didn't want.[5]

Are these uncommon or rare examples, or more the rule than the exception? They are common. The Associated Press reported that policies were cancelled for some 4.7 million people during the last weeks of 2013. The Obama administration became so worried about future hikes in premiums limiting signups on the exchanges that it gave insurers another year to meet the ACA's requirements.[6] While the exact number of cancellations is unknown, another estimate placed that number at about 2.6 million.[7]

The ACA did establish a number of needed requirements that private insurers were required to meet, including:

- Insurers must accept every individual who applies for coverage, regardless of pre-existing conditions.
- Prohibits insurers from imposing waiting periods.
- Requires insurers to vary rates only on four factors—family composition, geographic area, age, and tobacco use.

- Requires coverage of specified benefits in 10 categories of defined benefits: ambulatory patient services; emergency services; hospitalization; maternity and newborn care; mental health and substance use; prescription drugs; rehabilitative services; laboratory services; preventive and wellness services and chronic disease management; and pediatric services.
- Requires insurers to limit annual out-of-pocket costs.
- Requires insurers to cover at least 60 percent of total costs under each plan.
- Insurers must spend at least 80 to 85 percent of premium dollars on patient care.[8]

But concessions and delays to the insurance industry have left many insurers off the hook. As examples:

- Self-insured employer-sponsored plans are exempt from most of the ACA's requirements.
- As long as employers offer at least one plan that meets ACA's requirements, they are free to offer very lean "fixed-indemnity" plans that pay almost nothing toward the cost of a serious illness or accident.[9]
- Self-funded student health plans are exempt from annual and lifetime caps on benefits.
- High-deductible plans are held to lower standards.
- Insurers can exclude 70 percent of essential community providers from their networks.[10]
- In 2014, the Obama administration allowed plans that failed to meet the ACA's requirements in 2013 to be continued for two more years until 2016.[11]

Cancellations were still common in the fall of 2014, when Humana cancelled policies for more than 6,500 people in Kentucky and Kaiser Permanente dropped about 3,500 customers in the mid-Atlantic region. Other insurers cancelling policies included Baltimore-based CareFirst, Health Care Services Corporation in Chicago, and Golden Rule, a subsidiary of UnitedHealth Group.[12]

Insurers cancel for many reasons. The most common reason, of course, is that continuance of a plan that falls short of the ACA's requirements no longer makes business sense for the insurer. Most insurers are for-profit, with their highest priority the best return to shareholders. So they are quick to leave unprofitable markets. As one example, Blue Shield of California, which had just lost its state tax-exempt status with a surplus of more than $4 billion, withdrew from 250 zip codes throughout California in 2014.[13,14] As Ben Wakana, spokesman for the Department of Health and Human Services, readily acknowledges:

> *As was the case before the Affordable Care Act, private insurance companies operate in a free market: they may choose to discontinue, change and replace plans, so long as they let their enrollees know their options.*[15]

And, of course, insurers have always been free to cancel policies for an entire group, or to withdraw from the market entirely.

So, having looked at just one part of volatility in the private insurance markets, let's now turn our attention in the next chapter to another pervasive problem that seriously jeopardizes coverage for many millions of Americans—the constantly changing networks imposed by insurers.

References:

1. Adapted from Sundby, EL. You also can't keep your doctor. Commentary. *Wall Street Journal*, November 3, 2013.
2. Armour, S. Health costs hinge on high court ruling. *Wall Street Journal*, May 26, 2015: A1.
3. Ibid # 2.
4. Radnovsky, L, Mathews, AW. Some insurers cancel plans. *Wall Street Journal*, October 2, 2014: A3.
5. Stiffler, L. Health care improves in state, but could be better. *Seattle Times*, July 4, 2015.
6. Associated Press. Administration said to ponder insurance extension. *Business*, February 6, 2014.
7. Clemans-Cope, L. How many non-group policies were canceled? Estimates from December 2013. *Health Affairs Blog*, March 3, 2014.
8. Keith, K, Lucia, KW, Corlette, S. Implementing the Affordable Care Act: State action on the 2014 market reforms. *The Commonwealth Fund, February 2013.*
9. Centers for Medicare & Medicaid Services. Draft 2015 letter to issuers in the federally facilitated marketplaces, February 4, 2014.
10. Hancock, J. Insurers eye market for supplemental health coverage to fill gaps left by Obamacare, employer plans. *Kaiser Health News*, February 8, 2014.
11. Dennis, S. Administration extends Obamacare grandfathering for 2 more years. *Roll Call*, March 5, 2014.
12. Appleby, J. Cancelled health plans: round two. *Kaiser Health News*, October 2, 2014.
13. Terhune, C. With billions in the bank, Blue Shield of California loses its tax-exempt status. *Los Angeles Times*, March 18, 2015.
14. Bartolone, P. Capital Public Radio. Insurance choices dwindle in rural California as Blue Shield pulls back. *Kaiser Health News*, January 30, 2015.
15. Ibid # 5.

The Promise: If you are insured, your coverage (under the ACA) will be better and more secure than before.

CHAPTER 2

I HAVE INSURANCE, BUT MY NETWORK CHANGED

As we will see in more detail in Chapter 14, private insurers are taking advantage of their large new subsidized markets under the ACA as they compete in new ways for expanded market shares. One of these ways is to define (and redefine) which hospitals and physicians will be in their networks. They will tell us that they make these decisions on the basis of "quality," but that is typically a disingenuous claim. Their real motivation is to limit their costs by negotiating contracts with hospitals and physicians that are most favorable to the insurers themselves.

The ACA has been friendly to the insurance industry by permitting it to exclude a large proportion of hospitals and providers from their networks. The ACA initially required insurers to include just 20 percent of "essential community providers." However, a backlash soon broke out among hospitals and physicians on being arbitrarily excluded, forcing disruption of their established relationships with patients and breaking up continuity of care. In response, HHS proposed raising its requirement for government-run exchanges from 20 percent to 30 percent.[1]

Insurance networks are shrinking all across the country. A 2014 McKinsey report found that about 60 percent of health plans available through federal and state-run exchanges include a smaller number of hospitals than comparable current health plans. Some plans limit coverage to only one or two hospitals, in some cases excluding the only children's hospital or the major cancer care facility. A lawsuit has been filed in California by Santa Monica-based Consumer Watchdog against Cigna and Blue Cross of California over the size of their networks of doctors and hospitals, that end up leaving patients vulnerable to large out-of-network bills.[2]

Accountable care organizations (ACOs) are another key component of the ACA. In a theoretical effort to contain health care costs, they organize hospitals, other facilities, and providers into new arrangements that enable shifting from volume-oriented fee-for-service (FFS) reimbursement to a more comprehensive delivery of care and payment mechanisms. Hospitals and providers in each ACO contract to provide care for a population of at least 5,000 patients with the goal to achieve better coordination and quality of care at lower cost.

There are more than 500 ACOs around the country in various stages of development, more than half of which are for Medicare patients. ACOs add more confusion and disruption of care for many patients, since physicians may not know from quarter to quarter which of their patients are in their ACO and insurers can change networks at a moment's notice.

Impacts on Patients of Narrowed Networks

These patient vignettes illustrate some of the various circumstances that are such a problem for patients faced with changes of their insurance networks.

> *Bev Marcus and her husband had been insured by Premera Blue Cross on an individual policy that had covered most of his $150,000 bills for his heart attack and cancer care several years earlier. When they looked for a new policy with that insurer on Washington State's online insurance exchange for 2014, they found that none of the insurers' individual plans included any of Swedish's three*

hospitals in Seattle. If they stayed with Premera, they would pay much higher costs at out-of-network hospitals, while losing their cap for total out-of-network costs.[3]

Bob Rosenthal, 57-year-old former manager at a market-research firm in Los Angeles, purchased a top-tier "platinum" policy from Blue Shield of California for $792 a month, thinking that it would cover care at top hospitals. Several months later, he learned that the plan would not include the hospitals where he was used to being treated. As he said: "If I had anything happen, I wouldn't want to go to a hospital that I'm not familiar with and with doctors I don't know."[4]

Narrine Orange, in Florida, had the same problem as Bob Rosenthal. As she said: "I also picked the Platinum plan [with Blue Cross Blue Shield (BCBS)] and found out that my hospital and doctors were not covered. The best research I did before hand indicated that I would be covered and found after the fact that I was not. Got furious with BCBS and they agreed to correct a few cost items with my doctors. They are playing dollar games with our health and I am completely frustrated. I am not upset with Obamacare, only with the sly and sneaky insurance companies. Cannot drop my insurance and/or change until November of this year. What a fiasco. A single payer system would correct all of this smoke and mirror games played by the insurance industry."[5]

Peter Drier, 37-year-old bank technology manager in New York City, thought he was well prepared with insurance coverage for a three-hour neck surgery for herniated disks. He was blind-sided, however, when he received a bill for $117,000 from an out-of-network assistant surgeon he had never met. It is an increasingly common practice in hospitals and operating rooms across the country for assistants or consultants to be called in without the patient's *knowledge, who then bill the patient or the insurance company for their services. As Mr. Drier said: "I thought I understood the risks. But this was so wrong—I had no choice and no negotiating power."*[6]

Narrowed Networks: A System Problem Under the ACA

The above vignettes show how difficult it is for people to find out which hospitals and doctors are in their network. This is a built-in ongoing problem under the ACA as insurers, hospitals and physician groups negotiate and re-negotiate the terms of their contracts. Insurers are trying to get the lowest costs in order to offer lower premiums and attract more customers. Hospitals are trying to maximize their reimbursements, as are physician groups. Naturally, each of these three players has its own self-interest and business model in mind.

Although plans on the federal and state exchanges are required to include links to directories that show which hospitals and providers accept the insurance, much of that information is wrong. ZocDoc, an online appointment booking company, tried to verify the accuracy of hundreds of directories by calling doctors listed as in-network providers; about half the listings were wrong.[7] UnitedHealth Group, the largest plan of its kind with AARP's endorsement, planned to cut its national network of physicians by 10 to 15 percent by the end of 2014.[8] Many patients who get new coverage on the exchanges then find "phantom networks" of physicians who are incorrectly listed as network providers and will not accept them for care.[9] A 2014 study of physician directories publicized by Medicare Advantage plans found that only one-quarter of dermatologists listed would see new patients, and then only after a wait time of 45 days.[10] Many health plans sold through the exchanges in 2015 were so narrow as not to include such specialists as endocrinologists, rheumatologists, and psychiatrists; 15 percent of these plans did not include a single in-network physician in at least one specialty.[11]

As is obvious, patients are left at a disadvantage in trying to understand what hospitals and providers are in their networks. And these can change at any time, without much notice or recourse by insured patients. They often end up facing big bills from out-of-network providers, who may charge as much as 20 to 40 times the usual in-network rates. Unexpected out-of-network bills have become the leading complaint to the agency in New York State that regulates insurance companies, and efforts by other state regulatory agencies to limit patients' liability have been ineffective.[12]

All this is a replay of the managed care story in the 1990s, when patients' choices became so limited as HMOs expanded their markets. J. Mario Molina, CEO of Molina Healthcare Inc., a Long Beach, California-based managed care company ranked 301 in the Fortune 500, has this to say about the current situation:

> *This is the grand experiment. We're going to find out what consumers value more, choice or price.*[13]

But that is not the question! As this and the following chapters will show, we can probably agree that we as patients and our families value *both* choice and cost, and want much more say in our own health care than we have under the ACA.

References:

1. Wayne, A. Obamacare insurers may be forced to add medical providers. *Bloomberg Politics*, February 4, 2014.
2. Appleby, J. Consumer group sues 2 more Calif. plans over narrow networks. *Kaiser Health News*, September 25, 2014.
3. Landa, AS, Ostrom, CM. Many Wash. health-exchange plans exclude top hospitals from coverage. *Kaiser Health News*, December 3, 2013.
4. Tozzi, J. Obamacare limits choices under some plans. *Bloomberg Businessweek*, March 20, 2014.
5. Ibid # 4, comment.
6. Rosenthal, E. After surgery, surprise $117,000 medical bill from doctor he didn't know. *New York Times*, September 20, 2014.
7. Ibid # 4.
8. Cha, AE. Doctors cut from Medicare Advantage networks struggle with what to tell patients. *Health & Science*, January 25, 2014.
9. Terhune, C. Obamacare enrollees hit snags at doctors' offices. *Los Angeles Times*, February 4, 2014.
10. Resneck, JS Jr, Quiggle, A, Liu, M et al. The accuracy of dermatology network physician directories posted by Medicare Advantage health plans in an era of narrow networks. *JAMA Dermatology*, October 29, 2014.
11. Dorner, SC, Jacobs, DC, Sommers, BD. Adequacy of outpatient specialty care access in marketplace plans under the Affordable Care Act, *JAMA* 314 (16):1749, October 27, 2015.
12. Ibid # 6.
13. Martin, TW. Shrinking hospital networks greet health-care shoppers. *Wall Street Journal*, December 13-15, 2013: A4.

The Promise: If you are insured [under the ACA], your coverage will be more secure than before.

CHAPTER 3

I GOT INSURANCE, BUT THEN LOST IT

As we saw in the opening chapter, millions of Americans had health insurance before the ACA was enacted, but lost it for various reasons discussed there. But how stable is the insurance gained by the uninsured or previously insured when they get new plans through either the federal or state exchanges?

Before looking at that question, we need to acknowledge that some 16 million people have been successfully enrolled in these exchanges under the ACA, either through private plans or expanded Medicaid. This is, of course, a welcome development. But when we look more closely, this new coverage is frequently unstable, to the point that a new word has been added to our everyday vocabulary—"churning."

Despite promises by the Obama administration that you can keep your insurance if you like it, we find that assurance to be completely false.

Churning—Then and Now

Churning of health insurance coverage is by no means new, pre-dating the ACA for many years. Eligibility for private and public plans has long been in flux, depending on employment, income, age, geographical location, level of state participation in Medicaid, immigration status, and other factors. In more recent years, more employers have switched employees to part-time status in order to avoid providing them health insurance.

Discontinuity of health insurance coverage in this country has a long history. In 2003, for example, one study found that, over one three year period (1996-1999), 38 percent of all non-elderly Americans (85 million) were uninsured at any point in time.[1]

But the ACA has brought new complexities to eligibility and continuity of health insurance coverage. As Sara Rosenbaum, J.D. Professor of Health Law and Policy at the George Washington University School of Public Health and Health Services, observes:

> *The ACA introduces a new risk of churning for individuals and families whose income fluctuations mean they will move between Medicaid and subsidized private coverage through the marketplaces. The number of people likely to be in this situation is considerable: in a given year, half of those with incomes below twice the federal poverty level (FPL) can be expected to experience at least one income change sufficient to trigger movement from Medicaid to the marketplaces or vice versa.[2] This problem is likely to occur in all states—not only those expanding Medicaid—as enrollees' work, family, and life changes lead to movement across the three major public-subsidy programs (Medicaid, the Children's Health Insurance Program (CHIP), and the insurance marketplaces.[3]*

Here are three stories of how the ACA affected them, illustrating some of the problems in today's ACA marketplace for families and individuals:

> *Mark Segina and his wife, Jean, residents of Mount Vision, New York, were elated to get health insurance under the ACA after being uninsured for their entire adult lives. But the price was daunting: $360 a month to cover the two of them and their college-age son, after a subsidy of*

$777. Mark, 47, is a substitute teacher and high school coach whose work dries up in the summer. Jean, 42, is a dental hygienist. Their premium was their biggest monthly expense, higher than their mortgage payment. They have five children, ages 9 to 22. The younger children are insured through a state-subsidized program.

Every month, Mark and Jean talk about whether they could afford their MVP Health Plan another month. As soon as they got coverage, they went for checkups and other medical care they had deferred. Jean had a hernia operation that she had delayed for three years. As Mark said, 'We kind of felt like starving people that go to an all-you-can-eat buffet.' But after six months of coverage, they decided the expense was too great. They cancelled their policy and are back to being uninsured, although their oldest son is insured through his college. Mark voted for President Obama because he promised universal health coverage, but now feels the system established by the ACA is deeply flawed. As he says, 'by telling us we have to buy insurance, they basically have created a captive market. The insurers are going to charge what the market can bear and keep pushing the envelope until it collapses.'[4]

Alison Chavez, 36, who is self-employed, signed up for a marketplace plan in October 2013, hoping that it would be an improvement on her previous plan. With a new diagnosis of breast cancer, she was just beginning therapy, so was careful to choose a policy on the Covered California marketplace that included her physicians. But six months later, in the middle of treatment, she was notified that several of her doctors and the hospital were leaving the plan's network. She was forced to postpone a surgery and buy a new commercial policy that included her doctors. As she said, 'I've been through hell and back, but I came out alive and kicking, just broke.[5]

> *Stephanie Douglas, 50, working 30 hours a week as a dollar store cashier in Yazoo City, Mississippi and as a services coordinator at an apartment complex for older adults, signed up for health insurance through the federal exchange in January 2016. She had previously suffered a stroke and needed help paying for her care and medications. She qualified for subsidies, which cut her monthly payments to $58 a month. But that soon proved to be unaffordable, and she was forced to stop payments and lose her coverage several months later, saying "When you owe on your house, on your truck, when you're a single parent of a college student and you have other bills, it just doesn't work." [6]*

Since both public and private marketplace plans have their own, often changing, rules of eligibility and participation, churning will continue to be a major problem adversely impacting continuity and quality of care for enrollees.

Figure 3.1 summarizes income levels for eligibility for Medicaid, CHIP, and private qualified health plans. It includes most of our population, since premium tax credit eligibility under the ACA extends up to 400 percent of FPL ($46,680 for an individual, $95,400 for a family of four in 2015).[7]

When we look at the real numbers, churning will affect millions of people trying to navigate the shoals of unstable private and public plans. A recent study estimated that as many as 3.7 million nonelderly adults with coverage through state and federal exchanges will experience a "qualifying life event", (such as change in marital status, number of dependents, or loss of essential benefits) and become eligible for a special enrollment period because of income shifts in 2015. That study also found that more than 8.4 million nonelderly adults who did not have marketplace coverage (three of four without insurance) would have other qualifying life events that would make them eligible for subsidies in the private marketplace.[8]

FIGURE 3.1

PRODUCT MARKETS UNDER THE AFFORDABLE CARE ACT

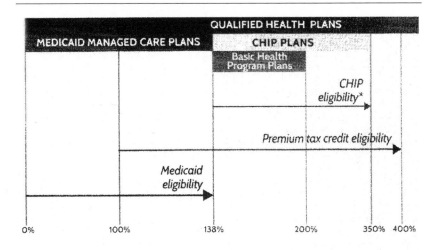

Percent of federal poverty level

* CHIP eligibility varies by state.

Source: Rosenbaum, S, Lopez, N. Dorley, M et al. Mitigating the effects of churning under the Affordable Care Act: lessons from Medicaid. *The Commonwealth Fund*, June 2014. Reprinted with permission.

Premiums are another key factor that change from year to year in the private marketplace. Most enrollees in 2014 chose a plan based on the monthly premium, often choosing the lowest premium with the greatest risk of losing continuity of care in narrow networks. Under the ACA, federal subsidies are tied to the benchmark silver plan (70 percent actuarial value). But the lowest cost silver plan may change from one year to the next. Caroline Pearson, vice president at Avalere, offers this advice to consumers:

> *The competitive landscape is changing in 2015 . . . the premium subsidies are tied to the benchmark plan and a percentage of income. Consumers have to pay the difference if they enroll in a plan more expensive than the benchmark. Those receiving federal premium subsidies may need to switch plans in 2015 to avoid paying more than the limits established by the ACA, and the impact will be more profound for lower-income consumers.*[9]

About 8 million people gained new insurance coverage after the first enrollment period under the ACA that ended in April 2014, 87 percent of whom were eligible for premium tax credits. But many faced confusion and uncertainty as to the tax refunds they could anticipate in 2015 as well as their premiums thereafter. Many would find their refunds delayed or less than expected, together with higher premiums in following years. Jon Kingsdale, Executive Director of the Commonwealth Health insurance Connector Authority in Boston, Massachusetts, and his co-author, Julia Lerche, further observe:

> *There is a high likelihood that the price and identity of the benchmark plan will change from year to year, as issuers adjust premiums, offer new, narrow network plans, enter new Marketplaces, and expand or contract service areas.*[10]

Looking at California as a case in point gives us further insight into the breadth and depth of the churning problem. Covered California, the state exchange, had to hire two outside firms in early 2014, at a cost of more than $13 million, to address the problem of long wait times for callers about their Obamacare coverage. A service-center staff of 1,300 was needed to help more than one million Californians renew their ACA coverage by January of 2015.[11] A study by the U.C. Berkeley Labor Center at that time showed that, in a 12 month period, one-fourth would leave Medi-Cal (the state's Medicaid program) and almost one-half would leave Covered California, while employer-sponsored plan enrollment would continually change.[12]

Given all the many factors that are changing each year for patients, their families, and insurers, churning will continue as a major barrier to continuity of coverage, which in turn relates to continuity and quality of care. The Urban Institute estimated that 9 million people would shift between Medicaid and the exchanges in 2014.[13] We can expect that instability to continue indefinitely, despite the massive bureaucracy trying to mitigate its adverse effects. As just one part in this growing bureaucracy, just imagine the burden on the IRS in having to track income levels that change every year in order to process tax credits and refunds for so many taxpayers.

Dr. Don McCanne, long-time family physician and health policy expert, sums up the problem this way:

> *Churning is inevitable in a model of health care financing that is fragmented between various private insurers and government programs, with varying eligibilities. If we had a single payer national health program—an improved version of Medicare that covered everyone—churning would not exist. It is too bad that our politicians and policymakers decided to cater to the interests of the private insurers than to meet the health care needs of the people. Maybe after enough people experience financial hardship and impaired access to care, the public will be ready for an improved Medicare for all.*[14]

References:

1. Short, PF, Graefe, DR, Schoen, C. Churn, churn, churn: how instability of health insurance shapes America's uninsured problem. Issue Brief. The *Commonwealth Fund*, November 2003.
2. Sommers, BD, Rosenbaum, S. Issues in health reform: how changes in eligibility may move millions back and forth between Medicaid and insurance exchanges. *Health Affairs* 30 (2): 228-236, February 2011.
3. Sommers, BD, Graves, K, Swartz et al. Medicaid and marketplace eligibility changes will occur often in all states: policy options can ease impact. *Health Affairs Web First*, March 2014.
4. Pear, R. Is the Affordable Care Act working? *New York Times*, April 26, 2014.
5. Rosenthal, E. Insured but not covered. *New York Times*, February 8, 2015.
6. Goodnough, A. Insurance dropouts present a challenge for health law. *New York Times*, October 11, 2015.
7. Rosenbaum, S, Lopez, N, Dorley, M et al. Mitigating the effects of churning under the Affordable Care Act: lessons from Medicaid. *The Commonwealth Fund*, June 2014.
8. Hartman, L, Espinosa, GA, Fried, B et al. Millions of Americans may be eligible for marketplace coverage outside open enrollment as a result of qualifying life events. *Health Affairs* 34 (5): 857-863, May 2015.
9. Carpenter, E. Exchange plan renewals: many consumers face sizable premium increases in 2015 unless they switch plans. Avalere, June 26, 2014.
10. Kingsdale, J, Lerche, J. An ounce of prevention for the ACA's second open enrollment. *Health Affairs Blog*, August 4, 2014.
11. Terhune, C. California spends $13.4 million to fix Obamacare service woes. *Los Angeles Times*, October 17, 2014.
12. Dietz, M et al. The ongoing importance of enrollment: churn in Covered California and Medi-Cal, April 2014. U. C. Berkeley Labor Center. http://laborcenter.berkeley.edu/healthcare/churn_enrollment.pdf
13. Bergal, J. Churning between Medicaid and exchanges could leave gaps in coverage, experts warn. *The Washington Post*, January 5, 2014.
14. McCanne, D. Churning in health care coverage. *Health Care Disconnects*. www.copernicus-healthcare.org/HCD.blogs/58.Churning.in.Health.Care.html

Promise: If you like your health care plan, you'll be able to keep your health care plan, period. . . . No one will take it away, no matter what.[1]

CHAPTER 4

MY EMPLOYER CUT BACK MY INSURANCE

Employer-sponsored health insurance (ESI) has a long history in this country. Its foundation was laid during the World War II years when three major forces came together—wage and price controls, worker shortages in a wartime economy, and strong unions. Corporations tended to enter into a long-term social contract with their employees by providing them with health insurance.[2] Because of that history, it is understandable that architects of the ACA included an employer mandate as a key part of its goal to expand insurance coverage. But as we will see, that policy was misguided, since ESI has been in long decline over many years. And President Obama's promises, stated above as a presidential candidate, were both naïve and deceptive.

The Steady Decline of Employer-Sponsored Insurance (ESI)

ESI as a social contract with employees is long gone, an archaic relic of the past. Fewer employers are offering health insurance, and when they do, more of the cost is being shifted to their employees. The economy has shifted from higher-wage unionized jobs with fringe benefits to lower-wage non-unionized service jobs with fewer or no benefits, with more workers unable to afford health insurance, even if offered. Moreover, an increasing proportion of the workforce works part-time, often in two or three part-time jobs, without any benefits at all.

By 2011, the proportion of nonelderly Americans with ESI fell to 58.3 percent, down from 69.2 percent in 2000. Coverage rates in that year varied widely by sector of the economy, ranging from 71.4 percent in the mining industry to 22.8 percent in the agriculture industry.[3]

The continued growth of costs of ESI has become more unaffordable for both employees and employers. The average cost of premiums for ESI employee-only coverage rose from $2,490 in 2000 to $5,081 in 2011, while family premiums increased from $6,415 to $14,447 in that same period.[4] Over the ten-year period from 2003 to 2013, average annual family premiums climbed by 73 percent, accounting for *23 percent of median family income*, up from 15 percent in 2003. Employers' contributions to these premiums increased by 93 percent over that period.[5]

An important 2015 article from the Center for American Progress called attention to "the great cost shift" from employers to employees, beginning well before the ACA, by which employers have shifted more responsibility for health care expenses to employees through higher deductibles, higher copayments, and higher coinsurance, as well as requiring them to pay a higher share of premiums.[6] A recent study found that deductibles for ESI plans have increased 67 percent since 2010, seven times the rise in workers' wages and general inflation.[7]

There are other problems with ESI. Job lock is an ongoing problem for many insured workers, who fear being unable to regain coverage if they change jobs. Even with ESI, there are still many reasons to feel insecure about continuing coverage, including if one loses his or her job, health status, income level (to afford rising costs), whether or not the insurer covers claims, and new caps on benefits.

The Employer Mandate under the ACA

The ACA sought to build upon ESI by requiring employers with 50 or more full-time equivalent employees who work 30 or more hours a week to offer health insurance to them by 2014 or pay a penalty of $2,000 for each full-time worker, excluding the first 30. That provision was later postponed to 2015 by the Obama administration, giving more time to work out the complex details of implementing this part of the legislation. Employers with 50-99 employees were allowed to delay meeting the ACA's requirements until 2016. Another requirement of the ACA was also relaxed for employers with 100 employees or more—they could avoid penalties in 2015 if they offered coverage to at least 70 percent of their full-time employees instead of the original 95 percent requirement.

Large employers, who generally retain control over costs and benefits of coverage by self-insuring, were exempted from most of the ACA's requirements with some exceptions They are required to cover preventive services without a lifetime or annual dollar value limit. And large employers offering high-cost group plans will face a 40 percent non-deductible excise tax on portions of total health insurance premiums above set levels starting in 2018 (the "Cadillac tax").

So how have employers responded to the employer mandate? Predictably, they have tried to get out from under this increasing burden in different ways, as these examples show:

- Walmart, the world's largest employer, dropped coverage in 2014 for 30,000 part-time employees who worked less than 30 hours a week; other big companies, such as Home Depot, Target, and Trader Joe's, have followed suit.[8]
- Many employers are shifting from defined benefit to a defined contribution system of just paying a certain amount toward their employees' coverage; others are dropping coverage or shifting employees to the exchanges.

- In order to keep their costs down, many employers are increasingly offering high-deductible plans, thereby shifting more costs to their employees.[9]
- Some employers with 50 or more employees are offering barebones "skinny" plans that cover preventive care but not such major benefits as hospital care.[10]
- As long as employers offer at least one plan that meets the ACA's requirements, they are free to keep offering others that do not, such as very bare bones "fixed indemnity" plans that pay almost nothing toward the cost of a major illness or accident.[11]
- Many small employers have cut workers' hours to less than 30 hours a week to get around the cost of insuring them.
- Some employers, especially those with lower-wage workers, such as in the food industry, have bypassed federal penalties by enrolling their employees in Medicaid plans.[12]
- In order to avoid the Cadillac tax, a growing proportion of large employers are moving to consumer-driven health care plans, with high deductible plans, which are held to a lower standard by the ACA, together with health savings accounts.[13]

Two-thirds of large employers expect that at least one of their health plans will be hit by the Cadillac tax in 2018, which applies to individual policies costing more than $10,200 a year and family policies over $27,500 a year. This is galvanizing a new coalition, The Alliance to Fight the 40, including major corporations, including Cigna and Pfizer, as well as union groups and other associations.[14]

Small business, the backbone of business in this country in terms of numbers and diversity, has its own special problems in dealing with the employer mandate. Compared to large employers, small employers lack the purchasing power to negotiate favorable rates with insurers. Here is a typical example that illustrates some of these problems:

*Aviva Starkman Williams, a California computer en-
gineer with employer-based insurance, tried to find out if
the pediatrician doing her 2-year-old's checkup was in the
plan's network for 2015. Only three of the pediatricians
in her doctor's six-person group were listed in her plan's
online directory. Since her deductible had tripled from the
previous year, she wanted to limit her out-of-pocket payments. The practice's office manager could not answer her
question. The insurer's representative said he also didn't
know, saying that doctors come in and out of the network
all the time.*[15]

Small business owners face challenging decisions about
whether to continue to offer ESI, what kind of policies to offer,
or drop coverage altogether. Here are two employers' dilemmas:

*Steven Laine, president and CEO of the 93-person
business consulting firm Future State, says that he could
make more money in the short term by cutting benefits, but
fears he would lose employees. The firm pays more than
50 percent of the premiums for 32 employees who take the
coverage it offers, costing about $200,000 a year. If all 77
full-timers were to participate in the plan the next year,
the firm's health care expenses would likely more than
double. But he doesn't know how many employees would
take up that plan. His insurance broker estimates that the
company's premiums would go up by 15 percent to 60
percent, regardless of how many employees join the plan.
If the company dropped coverage, it would face $94,000
in penalties and have difficulty in attracting or retaining
staffers without a health plan. As Mr. Laine says: "Moreover, dropping insurance fundamentally goes against our
organization's values."*[16]

*Chris Angelo is a second-generation owner of Stay
Green, a landscaping service in Santa Clarita, California, with 230 low-wage workers. Because of the ACA, the
firm plans to offer a health plan, but he is concerned that*

> *most workers will not be able to afford their share of the premiums. As Romerico Herrera, 48-year-old crewman making $11.50 an hour, said, "Of course, I prefer to have health insurance, because I need it for my children, for my family. I've had health insurance through previous employers, but not since working at Stay Green the last two years." Worried about the extent of coverage in the plan being offered, he wouldn't be able to pay more than $100 a month. As he said, "I make so little that [contributing] more would mean working just to pay for insurance."*[17]

The ACA set up a program intended to help small business owners to buy coverage for their employees, the Small Business Health Options Program (SHOP). By purchasing coverage for their employees through HealthCare.gov, employers with fewer than 25 employees that pay average annual salaries of $50,000 or less can qualify for tax credits worth up to 50 percent of their contribution toward their employees' premium costs. Although it is operational in 33 states, however, SHOP has received little interest from small employers.[18]

Do We Still Need Employer-Sponsored Insurance?

As we see from the above, what used to be, many years ago, a social contract between employers and employees, is in tatters. Both groups now find health insurance much too expensive. This situation has been building for a long time, and is not being redressed by the ACA. Moreover, many large companies are finding themselves less competitive in a global economy. As one example, a 2005 study found that General Motors was paying $1,500 per car for health insurance versus Canadian manufacturers across the river in Toronto paying little more than $200 per car and Toyota in Japan paying just $97.[19]

Economists have recognized the weaknesses of ESI for a long time. One such review highlighted its flaws in this way: "high administrative costs, inequitable sharing of costs, inability to cover large segments of the population, contribution to labor-management strife, and the inability of employers to act collectively to make health care more cost-effective."[20]

The ACA's employer mandate has not changed any of this for the better, leading us to conclude that ESI is no longer a rock to build upon.

Summary

As we have seen in earlier chapters, the ACA's dependence on the individual mandate has fallen way short of expectations. This chapter has shown the same for the employer mandate. As we have seen, ESI has been going downhill for many years, and was hardly a solid base to build on. Today, despite all attempts by the ACA, health coverage for employees so covered costs more for less coverage, is volatile from year to year, and often restricts choice of physician and hospital disrupting continuity and quality of care. When employees do take up ESI coverage, they tend to opt for plans with lower premiums and high deductibles that offer little protection against serious illness or accidents.

ESI has outlived its usefulness, is no longer affordable for employers or employees, limits choice, and makes business less competitive. The present situation with the ACA is untenable. We will look at options in Part Three.

References:

1. Drobnic Holan, A. "Lie of the year: If you like your health care plan, you can keep it." htpp://www.politifact.com/truth-o-meter/article/2013/dec/12/lie-of-the-year-if-you-like-your-health-plan-keep-it/). PolitiFact.com
2. Kuttner, R. The American health care system: Employer-sponsored health coverage. *N Engl J Med* 340: 248-252, 1999.
3. Gould, E. Employer-sponsored health insurance coverage continues to decline in a new decade. *Intl J Health Services* 43 (4): 603-638, 2013.
4. Robert Wood Johnson Foundation. Number of Americans obtaining health insurance through an employer declines steadily since 2000. Princeton, NJ, April 11, 2013.
5. Collins, SR, Radley, D, Schoen, C et al. National trends in the cost of employer health insurance coverage, 2003-2013. *The Commonwealth Fund*, December 9, 2014.
6. Spiro, T, Calsyn, M, O'Toole, M. The great cost shift: Why middle-class workers do not feel the health care spending slowdown. Center for American Progress, March 3, 2015.
7. News release. Employer family health premiums rise 4 percent to $17,545 in 2015, extending a decade-long trend of relatively moderate increases. *Kaiser 7. Family Foundation*, September 22, 2015.
8. Graham, DA. Walmart and the end of employer-based healthcare. *The Atlantic*, October 7, 2014.
9. Macdonald, J. Worried about insurance? That's common. *Bankrate.com*, September 4, 2014.
10. Hancock, J. Administration signals doubts about calculator permitting plans without hospital benefits. *Kaiser Health News*, October 18, 2014.
11. Centers of Medicare & Medicaid Services. Draft 2015 letter to issuers in the federally facilitated marketplaces, February 4, 2014.
12. Mathews, AW, Jargon, J. Firms try to escape health penalties. *Wall Street Journal*, October 22, 2014.
13. International Foundation of Employee Benefit Plans. 2015 Employer-Sponsored Health Care: ACA's Impact. May 15, 2015.
14. Abelson, R. Health care tax faces united opposition from labor and employers. *New York Times*, July 21, 2015.
15. Rosenthal, E. Insured but not covered. *New York Times*, February 8, 2015.
16. Maltby, E, Needleman, SE. Sizing up health costs. *Wall Street Journal*, May 30, 2013.
17. Maltby, E. The new math for health insurance costs. *Wall Street Journal*, June 7, 2013.
18. Janofsky, A. Small businesses spurn health exchanges. *Wall Street Journal*, January 8, 2015.
19. Taylor, M. Applying the brakes: UAW deal to affect providers as well as workers. (United Auto Workers union). *Modern Health Care* 35 (43):14, October 24, 2005.
20 Enthoven, AC, Fuchs, VR. Employment-based health insurance: past, present, and future. *Health Affairs* 25 (6): 1538-1547, 2006.

CHAPTER 5

I DON'T WANT OR NEED
HEALTH INSURANCE

In seeking to reduce the number of uninsured in this country, architects of the ACA hoped to broaden the risk pool in an effort to make insurance more efficient and affordable. Two basic mechanisms were employed—an individual mandate and an employer mandate. These concepts are actually a conservative approach, promoted in past years by the Heritage Foundation, and more recently implemented by Republican Governor Mitt Romney in the 2006 Massachusetts Health Act.

Now, having completed two full enrollment periods, we have enough evidence to assess how these mandates are working, as well as the extent to which they have reduced the numbers of the uninsured.

The Individual and Employer Mandates: Promises vs. Reality

There is strong evidence that the larger the risk pool, the more efficient and potentially affordable insurance can be. According to the National Institute for Health Care Management, 5 percent of the population accounts for one-half of health care spending, while 20 percent is responsible for 80 percent of that spending (the *20-80* rule).[1]

There were about 50 million Americans without health insurance in 2010, when the ACA was enacted. Although Barack Obama, as presidential candidate, promised to pass a bill for universal health coverage by the end of his first term in office, it was never designed to achieve universal coverage. Instead, the implicit message by its supporters was that it would gain near-full coverage.

The Individual Mandate

We are indebted to the Kaiser Family Foundation for its studies of the uninsured. It interviewed more than 10,000 individuals in the late fall of 2014, asking them to describe, in their own words, their experiences with the ACA's open enrollment process. There were many reasons for not getting insurance, as shown in Figure 5.1.[2]

FIGURE 5.1

REASONS BEING UNINSURED AMONG UNINSURED ADULTS, FALL 2014

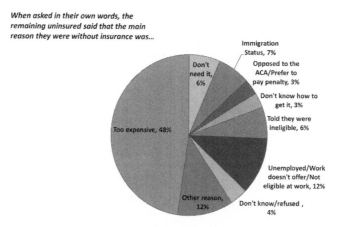

When asked in their own words, the remaining uninsured said that the main reason they were without insurance was...

Too expensive, 48%
Don't need it, 6%
Immigration Status, 7%
Opposed to the ACA/Prefer to pay penalty, 3%
Don't know how to get it, 3%
Told they were ineligible, 6%
Unemployed/Work doesn't offer/Not eligible at work, 12%
Don't know/refused , 4%
Other reason, 12%

NOTE: Includes uninsured adults ages 19-64.
SOURCE: 2014 Kaiser Survey of Low-Income Americans and the ACA.

Source: 2014 Kaiser Survey of Low-Income Americans and the ACA. Reprinted with permission.

By far the most common reason for staying uninsured is the unaffordability of insurance, despite the availability of subsidy/tax credits for people with annual incomes between 100 percent and 400 percent of FPL. Here are two typical patient experiences that illustrate the unaffordability of insurance:

> *Lisa Khechoom, 41, who runs a telecom-service business with her husband in Glendale, California, arranges for medical care through cash, barter or charity instead of buying health insurance. With their annual income of about $77,000, she asks "For the amount of office visits I do make, why pay $3,500 for insurance when I'm not even taking advantage of it? We go to the doctor and we pay for it. Usually I can get a better deal than if I had insurance."[3]*

> *Terrie Barlow, 64, in La Verne, California, is unemployed, hasn't had insurance for years, and pays for medical care out of pocket. She remains skeptical of the ACA, saying "I don't trust it. I don't see how it's affordable."[4]*

The penalty for not purchasing health insurance under the ACA's individual mandate in 2014 was $95 per adult or 1 percent of annual income, whichever was higher. But so many hardship exemptions were granted that only 90 percent of the almost 30 million uninsured would pay a penalty in that year.[5] There are 14 different categories of hardship exemption, including being homeless, filing for bankruptcy, and experiencing a death in the family.[6]

According to the IRS, the average penalty actually paid by 7.5 million people in 2014 was just $200.[7] But penalties for not having health insurance have since increased, as follows:

2015:	$325 per adult or 2 % of income
	$975 per family or 2 % of income
2016:	$695 per adult or 2.5 % of income
	$2,085 per family or 2.5 % of income

Some people choose to avoid insurance, even in the face of these penalties, as more cost-effective in their own circumstances, as this patient has done:

> *Beth Engel, 32-year-old mother of a three-year-old daughter, works part-time as a hotel clerk and qualifies for tax subsidies that would reduce premiums for her and her toddler to about $200 a month. An early supporter of the ACA, she now feels that the tax penalty for staying uninsured is much lower than paying for premiums. She has checked out plans offered by Covered California, the state exchange, but has decided to remain uninsured because of the high premiums. As she says, "Maybe I'm reading these incorrectly, but it just doesn't make sense, and I'm not going to put money I don't have into a program that I don't really understand."*[8]

Other patients have trouble with the ACA's coverage policies, as this patient describes:

> *A lot of AMA medicine is antiquated, and Obamacare doesn't pay for "alternative health care." In fact, using those alternative methods is what keeps me balanced and healthy, so I never need an M.D. My naturopath orders my blood work twice a year, and paying for all of that and all my prescriptions and supplements is still way less expensive than buying even the cheapest health care plan. Plus I get much better care. Why would I want to pay for a plan that doesn't provide good health care and is rigged so I will never get a benefit?*[9]

As we saw in Figure 5.1, there are still other reasons for not getting insurance. One of the biggest groups that remains uninsured includes those who would have been eligible for Medicaid had their states opted to accept federal funding to expand Medicaid. The ACA was intended to cover adults with incomes below the FPL and who are not disabled. But the U.S. Supreme Court left that decision up to the states, and more than 20 states opted out of that program. That resulted in almost 5 million adults falling into the "Medicaid coverage gap."

Many young adults choose not to get health insurance, in such numbers as to be labeled "young invincibles." At the close of 2014, one in five of the uninsured were young adults from 19 through 25 years of age.[10] Creatively, in an effort to "serve" this group, the insurance industry started marketing a "Young Invincibles" policy for young adults less than 30 years of age with an annual deductible of $5,950, indexed over time! It was not just younger people choosing to stay uninsured. A recent national study by Bankrate found that one-third of men between 50 and 64 years of age were also opting to remain uninsured.[11]

There are still other reasons for many people staying uninsured. Many who sought coverage under the ACA were told they were ineligible. Many were not aware of their options and lacked access to the Internet. Some found the process of exploring options too confusing. Others were opposed to being forced under government mandate to purchase insurance. Then there is the "family glitch"—the ACA was written in such a way that people who can afford their own coverage may find that coverage for other family members is too expensive, and those family members are not eligible for tax credits/subsidies.[12]

The Employer Mandate

As with the individual mandate, the employer mandate has been weakened under the ACA. Large employers were grandfathered in and exempted from the ACA's requirements. In response to the growing burden and expense of employer-sponsored insurance (ESI), many employers are shifting their employees to the exchanges, paying only a limited amount of the cost of insurance as a defined contribution, or dropping coverage altogether. ESI has become tenuous for many Americans. Millions of people gain, lose, or change their health insurance throughout the year, with many having to deal with long spells of not having coverage. Most who lost coverage in 2014 lost their employer-based coverage.[13] Figure 5.2 shows how little access employees had to ESI in 2014.

FIGURE 5.2

ACCESS TO EMPLOYER-SPONSORED INSURANCE AMONG UNINSURED ADULTS, FALL 2014

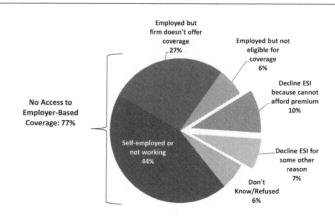

NOTE: Includes uninsured adults ages 19-64. Includes access to coverage through a spouse's job.
SOURCE: 2014 Kaiser Survey of Low-Income Americans and the ACA.

Source: 2014 Kaiser Survey of Low-Income Americans and the ACA. Reprinted with permission.

Summary

As a result of all these developments, both the individual and employer mandates have been seriously weakened, and are not able to expand the risk pool anywhere near what would be required to adequately share risk. Beyond that, of course, the ACA has given free rein to the private insurance industry to set their own prices and dominate expanded markets at taxpayers' ex-

pense. Professor Uwe Reinhardt, well-known health care economist at Princeton University, sums up the current predicament of
unaffordable health care costs this way:

> *One is inclined to put the blame mainly on the nation's
> business, health-industry and political leaders who over
> the past half century have joined forces to structure our
> health system so that U.S. health care now is twice as
> expensive on a per capita basis than health care in any
> other industrialized nation. Most of that differential can-
> not be explained by differences in the use of health care.
> It is driven mainly by much higher prices of health care in
> the U.S. These high costs of U.S. health care now make it
> politically difficult to provide families in the lower-middle
> income brackets more generous government subsidies
> than the ACA can offer.*[14]

We have to recognize the adverse impacts on so many Americans who still can't afford health insurance, forgo necessary care,
and have worse outcomes. The words of Gregg Bloch, M.D., J.D.,
Professor of Law at Georgetown University and author of *The
Hippocratic Myth: Why Doctors Are Under Pressure to Ration
Care, Practice Politics, and Compromise Their Promise to Heal,*
bring us back to the real issues:

> *At the heart of the case for medical coverage for all
> isn't the public's health; it's private tragedy. Serious ill-
> ness plunges people into a realm of Dickensian choice.
> Some forgo life-prolonging treatment to preserve life sav-
> ings for loved ones. Others lose their homes or go bank-
> rupt . . . Abandoning the sick to biology's random cruelty
> violates a widely-shared sense of decency. Caring, as an
> affirmation of our common humanity, inspired the quest
> for universal coverage.*[15]

So this and other chapters show how far we still are, despite "reforms" of the ACA, from the goal of universal coverage in this country. In the next chapter, we will look at what is happening with health insurance premiums.

References:

1. National Institute for Health Care Management. A comparatively small number of sick people account for most health care spending, August 2, 2012,
2. Garfield, R, Young, K. Adults who remained uninsured at the end of 2014. *Kaiser Family Foundation,* January 29, 2014.
3. Radnofsky, L. Meet the health-law holdouts. *Wall Street Journal*, June 25, 2015.
4. Armour, S, Radnofsky, L. Health-law sign-ups get tougher. *Wall Street Journal*, September 29, 2014.
5. Armour, S. Fewer uninsured face fines as health-law waivers swell. *Wall Street Journal*, August 7, 2014.
6. Young, J. What you need to know about Obamacare's individual mandate (and how much it costs to ignore it). *Huffington Post*, March 25, 2014.
7. Galewitz, P. Feds say 7.5 M paid an average penalty of $200 for not having health insurance. *Kaiser Health News*, July 21, 2015.
8. O'Neill, S, Southern California Public Radio. What Obamacare? Meet 4 people choosing to remain uninsured. *Kaiser Health News*, April 25, 2014.
9. Gerwick, M. Opinion/Letters, ACA holdouts, cost and employer- provided insurance. *Wall Street Journal*, July 6, 2015.
10. Ibid #2.
11. Flavelle, C. Obamacare's dropouts are middle-age men. *Bloomberg News*, March 17, 2014.
12. Rovner, J. Who is getting ACA insurance—and who isn't. *Kaiser Health News*, December 4, 2014.
13. Ibid # 9, p. 8.
14. Reinhardt, U. Letter to the editor. ACA holdouts, cost and employer-provided insurance. *Wall Street Journal*, July 6, 2015.
15. Bloche, G. Caring, freeloading, and the fate of the Affordable Care Act. *Health Affairs Blog*, September 19, 2012.

Promise by presidential candidate Obama: My health care reform bill will save the typical or average American family about $2,500 on their health insurance premiums.[1]

CHAPTER 6

I WANT INSURANCE, BUT CAN'T AFFORD THE PREMIUMS

The above promise amounts to one more untruth about what to expect with the ACA. It was not credible when made before the 2008 election, and experience since then has shown how far off it was.

We have seen how friendly the ACA is to the insurance industry. As examples, recall from Chapter 1 that self-insured employer-sponsored plans are exempt from most of the ACA's requirements, that high-deductible plans are held to lower standards, and that in 2014 the Obama administration allowed plans that failed to meet the ACA's requirements in 2013 could be continued until 2016. And since the U.S. Supreme Court upheld government subsidies for plans purchased through the exchanges, the industry will receive almost $2 trillion in ACA subsidies over 10 years through its expanded markets. After all this largesse from the ACA, we now look at how effective the ACA has been in making health insurance affordable.

The Continued Surge in Costs of Health Insurance

Since many of the requirements of the ACA had not kicked in for the first and second enrollment periods in 2013 and 2014, insurers had some latitude in setting premiums in the ACA's early years. They tended to keep initial premiums low in an effort to gain new enrollees. As many of us expected, premiums would likely increase later on, as we are now seeing.

When we look down the road, premiums will be even less affordable than encountered in the first years under the ACA, as indicated by these projections for 2016:[2]

- Blue Cross/Blue Shield plans, market leaders in many states, are seeking rate increases of 23 percent in Illinois, 25 percent in North Carolina, 31 percent in Oklahoma, 36 percent in Tennessee, 37 percent in Kansas, 51 percent in New Mexico, and 54 percent in Minnesota.
- The Scott & White plan in Texas has filed for a 32 percent rate increase.
- The Geisinger Health Plan in Pennsylvania has requested a 40 percent premium increase.
- The Arches Health Plan, which covers one-fourth of those who bought coverage through the federal exchange, requested a 45 percent rate increase.
- CareFirst plans, covering three-fourths of Maryland's residents who purchased plans on the state's exchange, will raise its average premiums 26 percent.[3]

Figure 6.1 shows other proposed average premium rates for 2016, together with how some were approved by state regulators.[4]

FIGURE 6.1

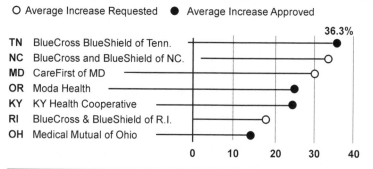

PROPOSED AND APPROVED
PREMIUM RATE INCREASES, 2016

Sources: Insurance filings submitted to state regulators; Radnofsky, L, Armour, S. Insurers win big health-rate increases. *Wall Street Journal*, August 27, 2015: A3.

Insurers defend these increases in various ways, including claims that enrollees were sicker than expected, that enrollees were older than anticipated, and that some costs were higher than expected, such as those for hospitalization, emergency room services, and specialty drugs.

But what they don't tell us are other ways that they actually prosper under the ACA beyond receiving pass-through subsidies from the government. As one example, the ACA includes a temporary federal "risk corridor" program from 2014 to 2016 that protects insurers from losses in qualified health plans sold in the individual and small group markets. Under this program, HHS provides payments to insurers that disproportionately attract higher-risk populations, such as individuals with chronic conditions.

Large insurers such as WellPoint (Anthem) and Humana expected to receive $5.5 billion in risk corridor payments in 2015.[5] Remember that the Obama administration *depends on* that participation for the ACA to work, and these risk corridor payments are one more way to keep insurers in the game.

How Affordable Are the Premiums?

Here are three vignettes showing how people of different circumstances and incomes found plans under the ACA unaffordable:

Wylene Gary, 40, an uninsured waitress in Yazoo City, Mississippi, tried to get health insurance through the federal exchange under the ACA, signed up and paid her first monthly premium of $129. But when her new insurance card came in the mail, she was shocked to find that it had a $6,000 deductible and 40 percent co-pay. She called the representative for the insurer, Magnolia Health, asking whether the co-pay meant that she would have to pay $40,000 if she incurred a $100,000 bill. The answer was "yes." She was not told that her out-of-pocket costs would be legally capped at $6,350, and she cancelled her coverage.[6]

Steven Peterson, 40, manages a health store in West Hollywood, California. He is uninsured, and plans to stay that way because of the cost of insurance. The lowest premium he could find on the exchange was $240 a month. As he says, "I'm a pretty healthy guy, so I really don't see the point of it because it's so expensive." He would rather have an inexpensive catastrophic coverage plan, but those are only offered to consumers under 30 years of age or people with hardship exemptions.[7]

Michael Kole, 52-year-old sales and marketing entrepreneur, earns too much to qualify for government subsidies for health plans purchased through the federal insurance exchange. After the ACA kicked in, his monthly premiums for coverage of himself and his family went up from $513 to $848 ($10,176 a year). He wasn't happy about that, saying "It's taking a lot out of pocket." To save money, he now works from home instead of renting an office.[8]

Gunnar Ebbesson, a small business owner with a family of five in Fairbanks, Alaska, could not afford a 2016 premium hike to more than $40,000 a year for his Premera policy, a barebones plan with a $10,000 deductible. With an annual income more than $142,000, he was not eligible for subsidies, and was forced to cancel his coverage. (Alaska has the highest health insurance rates in the country, with an average annual premium of more than $8,600 for a 40-year-old in Anchorage).[9]

The Commonwealth Fund has defined these helpful markers for *under*insurance: "People who are insured all year, but report at least one of these three indicators: (1) medical expenses amounting to 10 percent or more of annual income; (2) among low-income adults below 200 percent of FPL, medical expenses at or more than 5 percent of income; and (3) health plan deductibles at or more than 5 percent of income."[10] But a recent study, again by the Commonwealth Fund, has found that almost 10 percent of median household income already goes to insurance premiums and deductibles, *not including other cost-sharing requirements, such as co-insurance and co-pays, and other out-of-pocket expenses for health care actually received.*[11] Moreover, Pew Charitable Trusts have shown that 55 percent of American households are savings-limited, able only to replace less than one month of their income through liquid savings.[12]

The median household income in the U.S. was $53,657 in 2014, down from $57, 357 before the recession and its peak of $57,843 in 1999, according to the latest data available by Census data.[13] Yet more than $5,000 is being spent, *just for insurance*, without all of the other costs of health care. In 2014, according to the 2014 Milliman Medical Index (MMI), total health care costs, including insurance, for a typical family of four with employer-sponsored health insurance, came to $23,215, including payroll deductions and out-of-pocket costs. Over the ten-year period from 2004 to 2014, the MMI grew by an average of 7.6 percent a year, about three times the annual growth rate of the consumer price index (CPI of 2.3 percent).[14] By the fall of 2015, among adults age 19-64 visiting the ACA's exchanges, 57 percent could not afford a plan.[15] So private health insurance has already priced itself beyond the means of much of the population, but survives through the ACA's subsidized markets and employers' contributions to employer-sponsored plans.

Can Premiums Be Reined in by Regulators?

Regulation of the private insurance industry has historically been ceded by the federal government to the states. The insurance markets in states are complex, vary widely from one state to another, and are divided into three big groups—large group, small group, and individual—thereby resulting in 150 different state-level markets. The insurance lobby has been extremely strong in state houses across the country for many years, and has been generally able to avoid significant regulation of premiums.

The state of Oregon gives us a bellwether of what we can expect from state regulation of premiums under the ACA. Despite being a relatively liberal state, the Oregon insurance commissioner called for *increases* of premium rates by an average of 34.8 percent for Health Net (which had requested a 9 percent hike) and 19.9 percent for Oregon's Health Co-op (compared to its 5.3 percent increase request). After public hearings and a rigorous review, the commissioner, an actuary, found that premium income in 2014 was $703 million, far short of the $830 million paid out to individuals and families for their care. She defended these increases over a concern that "inadequate rates could result in companies going out of business in the middle of the plan year, or being unable to pay claims."[16] So, based on this example and the long-standing weakness of state regulation of premiums, we can anticipate that premiums will be increasingly unaffordable.

The ACA itself has deemed premiums for ESI coverage affordable if they are no more than 9.5 percent of family income. When we consider that premiums do not cover other cost-sharing and out-of-pocket costs, health care obviously becomes unaffordable for many millions of people, as we shall see in more detail in Chapter 11.

There is now a battle going on behind the scenes between insurers, analysts, and policymakers about how to deal with the growing unaffordability of health insurance. One long-term analyst of the ACA, Robert Laszewski, president of Washington-based Health Policy and Strategy Associates, LLC, has warned for some years that a large sustainable risk pool is critical to the ACA's success. But that has not happened, as he points out in a recent article. After two open-enrollment periods, we have low take-up rates by those eligible for the exchange market across the country, as these examples show: Kansas (less than 40 percent), Maryland (30 percent), Oregon (35 percent), Pennsylvania (50 percent), and Tennessee (less than 40 percent).[17]

It has now become clear that there are not enough healthier people enrolled in the exchanges to avoid adverse risk in the insurance markets. That problem is made worse by the large numbers of people who would rather pay the penalties than buy coverage with less and less value. Going for the lowest premiums usually requires patients to accept narrower networks of hospitals and physicians, with disruption of continuity of care. Summing up this fundamental problem, Laszewski makes this blunt assessment:

> *[Forcing people to change plans in order to avoid huge premium increases is just one problem of many]. . . . This is a debacle. This is a blow-up. This is a mess. There's big trouble in Obamacare land. The biggest carriers are losing their shirts and thus seeking the biggest rate increases.*[18]

As we recall from the last chapter, 5 percent of the population accounts for 50 percent of health care spending, with 20 percent accounting for 80 percent of these costs. The bigger the risk pool, the more efficient health insurance can be in spreading risks. As they deal with expanding markets under the ACA, insurers try not to expand into populations that increase their exposure to sick people. When asked about his company's strategy in adjusting to the ACA, Mark Bertolini, Aetna's CEO, has said that "We are very careful to pick the markets."[19]

Faced with a gathering firestorm over the cost and value of private health insurance, HHS has issued an appeal to state insurance commissioners to give insurer rate requests more scrutiny, but this appeal is likely to be ineffective as the insurers continue to raise rates for products of decreasing value to enrollees. With this latest appeal, HHS also tried to reassure insurers that they can expect to receive additional special federal payments if needed to continue at-risk health plans through 2016.[20]

Summary

How could we have expected a for-profit private insurance industry to rein in its costs of premiums in a supposedly competitive environment when the opportunity to exploit expanded new subsidized markets was handed to them? Its game now is to offer plans at higher premiums, with less and less coverage, as we will see more in Chapter 10. As the industry thrives, at patients' and taxpayer expense, it is stronger and more powerful than ever, controlling more of how health care is delivered.

This situation raises two questions. Have insurers that dominate the market become too big to fail, as we have let the banks become? And as the government continues to favor the insurance industry over the needs of patients and their families, who is the patient—the industry or real people? We will return to these questions in Part Three of this book.

References:

1. Wogan, JB. No cut in premiums for typical family. The Obameter. PolitiFact, August 31, 2012.
2. Pear, R. Health insurance companies seek big rate increases for 2016. *New York Times*, July 3, 2015.
3. Goldstein, A. Price to jump for most popular health plan on Maryland insurance exchange. *The Washington Post*, September 4, 2015.
4. Radnofsky, L, Armour, S. Insurers win big health-rate increases. *Wall Street Journal*, August 27, 2015: A3
5. Wayne, A. Insurers' Obamacare losses may reach $5.5 billion in 2015. *Bloomberg News Businessweek*, March 4, 3014.
6. Varney, S. In the country's unhealthiest state, the failure of Obamacare is a group effort. *Kaiser Health News*, October 29, 2014.
7. Ibid # 6.
8. O'Neill, S. What Obamacare? Meet 4 people choosing to remain uninsured. Southern California Public Radio. *Kaiser Health News*, April 25, 2014.
9. Feidt, A. Alaskans face tough choices because of high insurance costs. Alaska Public Radio Network. *Kaiser Health News*, October 30, 2015.
10. Schoen, C, Doty, M, Collins, SR et al. Commonwealth Fund. Insured but not protected: How many adults are underinsured, the experiences of adults with inadequate coverage mirror those of their uninsured peers, especially among the chronically ill. *Health Affairs Web Exclusive*, June 14, 2005.
11. Rosenthal, E. Insured, but not covered. *New York Times*, February 8, 2015.
12. Pew Charitable Trusts. The precarious state of family balance sheets. January 29, 2015.
13. 2014 Census ACA Data. Department of Numbers. Washington, D.C. http://www.deptofnumbers.com/income/us/
14. Armour, S. Health costs hinge on Supreme Court's ruling. *Wall Street Journal*, May 25, 2015.
15. Collins, SR, Gunja, M, Dotie, MM et al. To enroll or not to enroll? Why many Americans have gained insurance under the Affordable Care Act while others have not. *The Commonwealth Fund*, September 25, 2015.
16. Ibid # 2.
17. Laszewski, R. Why are the 2016 Obamacare rate increases so large? *Forbes Opinion*, June 10, 2015.
18. Rovner, J. HHS pushes states to negotiate lower Obamacare rates. *Kaiser Health News*, July 22, 2015.
19. Bertolini, M. As quoted by Martin, TW, Weaver, C. For many, few health-plan choices, high premiums on online exchanges. *Wall Street Journal*, February 12, 2014.
20. Ibid # 19.

CHAPTER 7

MEDICAID HASN'T HELPED ME

Since its passage in 1965, Medicaid has been a vital part of what safety net we have in health care around the country. From the start, it has been jointly funded by the federal government and the states, with their respective shares varying over the years. It has served as a last resort for health care coverage for many millions of Americans, and since the 1990s has become the main payer for nursing home care. It was only natural that those shaping the ACA would build expansion of access to care around Medicaid's long established role. The ACA therefore provided 100 percent federal funding for the first three years to states to expand their programs; that would later phase down to a 90 percent federal share by 2020. In addition, higher reimbursement for primary care physicians was built into the law on a temporary basis to help with access to care.

Now, almost six years after enactment of the ACA, we will examine the extent to which Medicaid has met its goals.

The ACA and Medicaid—A Mixed but Unacceptable Record

There is no question but that expansion of Medicaid under the ACA has made a big positive difference for millions of Americans in need of necessary health care. The uninsured rate for people in poverty soon dropped from 28 percent to 17 percent in states that expanded Medicaid. But after the U. S. Supreme Court ruled in 2012 that states could choose whether or not to expand Medicaid, more than 20 states opted out. As a result, while the uninsured rate for people in poverty dropped from 28 percent to 17 percent in states that expanded Medicaid, it fell by only 38 to 36 percent in non-expanding states.[1]

With post-ACA added enrollments in Medicaid, the program today covers about 70 million people, including low-income adults under age 65, almost one-half of all births, one-third of children, two-thirds of people in nursing homes, and the disabled. As a federal-state hybrid, states have considerable flexibility to set their own eligibility and coverage rules.[2]

Despite important gains in access to care, there are still many ways in which Medicaid falls short of our needs, some of which are systemic problems that pre-dated the ACA. Here we consider the main ones.

States opting out

More than 20 states opted out of expanding Medicaid under the ACA, mostly in red states in the South. But some states, even including some opt-out states, still welcome federal money, which they then use to contract out to private insurers under Medicaid managed care (MMC), with the belief that they will be more efficient.

As a result of the Supreme Court's decision, a "Medicaid coverage gap" was created whereby almost 5 million people are ineligible for Medicaid because of incomes below the federal poverty level (FPL) but above Medicaid eligibility levels. Here are two examples of patients falling into this gap through no fault of their own:

> *Greg Morris, 46, a single father in Osage County, Missouri, works part-time at a miniature golf course. He is one of about 300,000 Missouri residents in the Medicaid coverage gap. As he says, "The only option I have is to pay more than I can afford. I wish they would go ahead and expand the Medicaid the way the law was designed."*[3]

> *Charlene Dill was a 32-year-old mother of three who earned $11,000 a year cleaning houses and babysitting in Florida. That was too much to qualify for Medicaid and too little to afford health insurance. The ACA would have provided subsidies for health insurance if her income was more than $23,550. When she developed a heart condition, and later, abscess on her legs, she did go to emergency rooms, but couldn't afford those bills or any other care. She died of treatable conditions because Rick Scott, the multimillionaire governor with a long track record of fraud with HCA, the giant hospital chain, refused to accept federal Medicaid expansion money under the ACA.[4]*

Unfortunately, the above story is not an isolated case. A recent study estimates that at least 7,100 people will die without Medicaid coverage in non-expanding states.[5] Another recent study by the Commonwealth Fund found that more than 40 percent of residents in Texas and Florida reported not going to a doctor when they were sick, filling a prescription, seeing a needed specialist, or skipped a recommended test or treatment in the previous year.[6]

Variable eligibility

Eligibility for Medicaid varies widely from one state to another, as these unfortunately common patient experiences illustrate:

> *Jasmin Harrison, 23, was insured up until a year previously as a nurse's assistant. But after a driver rear-ended her, she developed debilitating pain and couldn't keep up her shifts. She then had about $40,000 in medical bills, no job and no insurance. She tried to sign up for coverage on the exchange, but fell into the Medicaid coverage gap. A counselor told her that she was ineligible because she had no income, and that she would have to get pregnant or have children to become eligible.[7]*

Tamasha Fields, a 27-year-old mother of a four year-old son, has an annual income of about $7,000 with a cleaning service in Alabama. She presented to the University of Alabama's Hospital in Birmingham for treatment of a miscarriage. She earned too much to be eligible for Medicaid in Alabama, where the income ceiling is just $2,832 for a family of two, after deductions.[8]

Teresa Stoikes, a 58-year-old Missouri native, moved back to the state looking for work in 2002, but has been unable to find a full-time job. She has no health insurance. She would qualify for Medicaid if the state expanded eligibility. Her income is about $465 a month, $5,580 a year, from a pension. But she was turned down for Medicaid because she does not fit any of the traditional eligibility categories: she does not have a disability, is not over the age of 64, and does not have dependent children. She lives near Fort Leonard Wood in the Missouri Ozarks, and has diabetes that has caused eye and kidney problems. But she makes too little to qualify for financial assistance through the ACA. Those subsidies are available for people with incomes from 138 percent to 400 percent of the FPL, but not below the poverty level. She has been taking insulin and metformin, an oral diabetes drug, but has been hospitalized several times. She now has thousands of dollars in medical debt, wants to avoid more debt, but is trying to figure out how to get needed eye surgery. As she says, 'If I am allowed to get on Medicaid, I will definitely do it. If I were on Medicaid, I would not have to be afraid of going to the hospital if I needed to. Now, I have to ask myself, is what's happening serious enough to go to a doctor or hospital?'[9]

Financial Barriers

Some states have received federal waivers to impose premiums and/or copays on Medicaid patients. This cost sharing has been shown to result in disenrollment and decreased access to care.[10]

Unavailability of Doctors

Getting coverage under Medicaid does not in any way assure access to care. A 2015 study by HealthPocket found that only one-third of U.S. physicians are accepting Medicaid patients. Typical Medicaid reimbursement is just 61 percent of what Medicare pays for the same service. The ACA attempted to address this problem by temporarily increasing primary care reimbursement to Medicare levels in 2013 and 2014. But a study by the nonpartisan Urban Institute estimated that primary care physicians would have their reimbursements cut by an average of 43 percent after 2014.[11] Meanwhile, an increasing number of states have been moving away from fee-for-service (FFS) reimbursement and have moved many or all of their Medicaid patients into mostly for-profit managed care programs, with reimbursement through pre-set capitation payments based on the total number of patients in the plan.[12] The capacities of their networks are highly variable, from 750 patients per doctor in Michigan to 2,500 per doctor in Tennessee.[13]

State directories of physicians supposedly accepting Medicaid patients are inaccurate and unreliable. As one example, four in ten physicians listed in California's Medicaid (MediCal) directory in 2014 were either unavailable to new patients or could not be reached.[14] As a result of restricted access to primary care, emergency room visits have increased, not decreased, as was the ACA's original hope.[15]

Inadequate Coverage

Since states have wide latitude to set their own coverage policies, big deficits in what we would call essential care have long been a problem with Medicaid. Under the ACA, as with eligibility, Medicaid coverage remains highly variable from one state to another. As one example, the ACA requires expanded Medicaid to cover the U.S. Preventive Services Task Force's A- and B-rated services without cost sharing; this is the scientific body that makes recommendations based on best evidence for or against screening procedures. These include screening for hypertension, diabetes, depression, and cancer. But Medicaid programs in many states still do not cover these basic services, while confusion continues over what services will be covered in any one state.[16]

Privatized Medicaid

More than one-half of Medicaid patients are now in privatized Medicaid managed care plans (MMC). But that does not mean that they have good access to physicians. Each privatized MMC program lists large numbers of physicians in its network. But these are often "phantom networks." A 2014 report from the Inspector General of the Department of Health and Human Services, based on a study of 1,800 providers and more than 200 health plans in 32 states, found that more than one-third of providers could not be found at the location listed by the MMC plan, that 8 percent were at the listed location but were not participating in the plan, and that another 8 percent were not accepting new Medicaid patients. When appointments were offered, the median wait time was two weeks, with one-quarter of appointments delayed by more than one month.[17]

MMC health plans are paid on a capitation basis, a set negotiated rate to cover all of their enrollees' medical needs. Based on their for-profit status and business model, they are incentivized to limit access, choice, and services. Many of these plans have inadequate physician networks, long waits for care, denials of many treatments, and poor accountability for quality of care. How can anyone justify this example of an inhumane coverage decision in a Kentucky MMC?

Kaden Stone was just 3 feet 6 inches tall and 48 pounds at age 8 because of congenital bowel problems that have required dozens of surgeries and procedures. He relied on PediaSure, an expensive nutritional drink, for sustenance

*until his private Medicaid plan stopped paying for it, call-
ing it not medically necessary.*[18]

So far we have no evidence that MMC improves health care
outcomes. The record to date is mixed, but concerning. A 2015
study by the Urban Institute found that increased penetration of
MMC plans is associated with increased probability of an emergency room visit, difficulty in seeing a specialist, and unmet need
for prescription drugs; the investigators concluded that 'This sug-
gests that the primary gains from MMC may be administrative
simplicity and budget predictability for states rather than reduced
expenditures or improved access for individuals.'[19]

The Future of Medicaid

Although Medicaid now covers almost one in four Americans, it is far from an adequate safety net, as we have just seen. As
it moves steadily toward for-profit privatized MMC plans, we can
expect more restricted access, choice, and quality of care, as well
as increased administrative costs with profiteering at the expense
of the needs of patients and their families. As a 2015 article points
out, its future challenges will fall into five areas: (1) controlling
costs; (2) getting states to expand income eligibility under the
ACA; (3) better oversight of managed care; (4) ensuring access
to doctors; and (5) meeting the growing demand for long-term
care.[20]

Medicaid continues to be treated as an underfunded welfare
program. It is greatly limited by the lack of standards for access
and quality of care. Wide variations from state to state compromise its reliability as a safety net. Its surge in enrollment under
the ACA has brought higher costs to many states than expected as
states struggle against declining tax revenues. A 2015 review by
Associated Press found at least 22 states to be facing budget shortfalls for the 2016 fiscal year.[21] In this environment, Medicaid is

under constant threat politically for draconian cuts in many states, especially those in the South and interior Midwest.

The future of Medicaid goes to the heart of the larger debate over financing of U.S. health care. As health care becomes ever more unaffordable for an increasing part of our population, the urgency of a national approach grows. In Part Three we will consider three major options going forward.

References:

1. Collins, SR, Rasmussen, PW, Doty, MM. Gaining ground: Americans' health insurance coverage and access to care after the Affordable Care Act's first open enrollment. *The Commonwealth Fund*, July 10, 2014.
2. Galewitz, P. 5 challenges facing Medicaid at 50. *Kaiser Health News*, July 27, 2015.
3. Appleby, J, Gorman, A. Obamacare enrollment: second year even tougher. *Kaiser Health News*, October 6, 2014.
4. Dispatches. Working mother dies of medical neglect in Florida. *The Progressive Populist*, April 15, 2014.
5. Dickman, SL, Himmelstein, DU, McCormick, D et al. Health and financial harms of 25 states' decision to opt out of Medicaid. *Health Affairs Blog*, January 30, 2014.
6. Rasmussen, P, Collins, S, Doty, M et al. Health Care Coverage and Access in the Nation's Four Largest States. Results from the Commonwealth Fund Biennial Health Insurance Survey, 2014. *The Commonwealth Fund*, April 10, 2015.
7. Varney, S. In the country's unhealthiest state, the failure of Obamacare is a group effort. *Kaiser Health News*, October 29, 2014.
8. Weaver, C. Millions trapped in health-law coverage gap. *Wall Street Journal*, February 10, 2014: A1.
9. Pear, R. Is the Affordable Care Act working. *New York Times,* April 26, 2014.
10. Dickson, V. Medicaid cost-sharing could reduce enrollment, experts warn. *Modern Healthcare*, September 16, 2014.
11. Pear, R. As Medicaid rolls swell, cuts in payments to doctors threaten access to care. *New York Times*, December 27, 2014.

12. Smith, VK, Gifford, K, Ellis, E et al. Medicaid in an era of health & delivery system reform: results from a 50-state Medicaid budget survey for state fiscal years 2014 and 2015. *Kaiser Family Foundation*, October 14, 2014.

13. Bergal, J. Advocates urge more government oversight of Medicaid managed care. *Kaiser Health News*, July 5, 2013.

14. Guzic, H. Directories of doctors who treat the poor are inaccurate, hurting access. *California Health Report*, June 29, 2014.

15. Tavernise, S. Emergency visits seen increasing with health law. *New York Times*, January 2, 2014.

16. Wilensky, SE, Gray, EA. Existing Medicaid beneficiaries left off the Affordable Care Act's bandwagon. *Health Affairs* 32 (7): 1188-1195, 2013.

17. Pear, R. Half of doctors listed as serving Medicaid patients are unavailable, investigation finds. *New York Times*, December 8, 2014.

18. Bergal, J. Kentucky's rush into Medicaid managed care: a cautionary tale for other states. *Kaiser Health News*, July 18, 2013.

19. Caswell, KL, Long, SK. The expanding role of managed care in the Medicaid program. *Inquiry*, April 16, 2015.

20. Ibid # 2.

21. Associated Press. Medicaid enrollment surges, stirs worry about state budgets. July 19, 2015.

Promise: If you like your doctor, you will be able to keep your doctor.[1]

CHAPTER 8

I HAVE INSURANCE, BUT LOST MY DOCTOR

As we have seen in earlier chapters, patients seeking insurance coverage through the ACA's exchanges tend to select plans with the lowest premiums, often not realizing the trade-offs that result. It has become so commonplace as to become a new norm for millions of the newly insured, as well as those who had their previous policies cancelled, that they lose their doctor along the way. This seriously disrupts continuity and compromises quality of care.

Here we will look at five major systemic changes, some predating but all exacerbated by the ACA, that have made this new norm a reality for too many people.

System Changes Disrupting Continuity of Care

1. Accountable care organizations and changing networks

Three major trends in the U.S. health care system have been accelerated by the ACA—(1) the growing role of accountable care organizations (ACOs); (2) consolidation of hospital systems, typically taking ownership of large physician groups; and (3) the narrowing of insurance networks as insurers compete by trying to lower costs by including lower-cost providers. These two examples show how big the impacts can be on large numbers of patients:

- UnitedHealthGroup Inc, the biggest player in the Medicare Advantage market with almost 3 million enrollees and 350,000 physicians in its networks, dropped thousands of physicians from its networks in at least ten states in the last months of 2013; about 2,500 cancer patients at Moffitt Cancer Center in Tampa, Florida, were forced to switch plans or find other physicians.[2]
- Also in late 2013, the University of Pittsburgh Medical Center (UPMC) sent certified letters to several hundred patients informing them that they could no longer see their physicians. This was because their insurance, Community Blue, sold by Highmark, had become both a rival hospital system and an insurer. Some cancer patients were cut off from their UPMC physicians in the middle of their treatments.[3]

Here is one patient's story in trying to deal with these kinds of changes:

> *Amy Moses, a tech entrepreneur in New York City, selected a health plan on line with the goal to keep her longtime physician. She paid $650 per month for a United Healthcare plan that did include that physician. Not long later, the doctor's practice was bought by a hospital, which then dropped the plan, as did her doctor (though he was still listed in the directory a year later!). She only discovered this change when she contacted her doctor to request a referral for an urgent outpatient procedure costing thousands of dollars that had been recommended by an in-network surgeon. (Both the referring physician and the surgeon had to be in-network for coverage). As she said, 'I literally had three days to find a new in-network internist, get an appointment to make the referral, or cancel the procedure. I was stuck in insurance purgatory.[4]*

2. Narrow networks

There is an ongoing battle between insurers and regulators as to what constitutes an adequate network of hospitals and physicians. Insurers want the smallest network with the lowest cost providers, without much regard for quality of care and with no concern for continuity of care. Federal guidelines are still loose, so far allowing insurers to include only 30 percent of "essential community providers" in their networks. Not only are networks shrinking across the country, but they can also change at a moment's notice.

This patient illustrates these problems:

Karen Pineman, 46, self-employed in Manhattan, New York, had her long-time health insurance policy cancelled for not meeting the ACA's requirements. She purchased new Blue Cross/Blue Shield coverage through the exchange, accepting that she would have to pay out-of-pocket for her primary care physician, who was not in the plan's network. When she broke her ankle playing tennis, she had co-pays of almost $1,800 to have a cast put on her ankle in an emergency room. When she tried to arrange a follow-up appointment with an in-network orthopedist, the insurer said that the nearest available orthopedist was in Stamford, Connecticut, 14 miles away. Then on crutches, she protested and was told that as much as 15 miles was considered a reasonable travel distance. Instead, she paid $350 to see a nearby orthopedist and buy a boot at his recommendation. Since then she paid hundreds of dollars more for a physical therapist who was in-network but not covered by the plan.[5]

3. Lack of information

The inaccuracy of directories of physicians supposedly available within insurers' networks has become so pervasive as to be a major problem for patients seeking to keep their care in-network for continuity and cost reasons. This patient's story, unfortunately, is all too typical:

> *Dr. Alexis Gersten, a dentist in Eact Quoque, New York, switched her family and 11 employees to a new Blue Cross/Blue Shield plan for 2014, after her previous small business group plan was canceled. She purchased the new plan through a broker, and was unaware that it was an ACA plan. When her son needed an ear, nose and throat specialist, the nearest was in Albany, five hours away. Though her cardiologist was on the network list, he said he did not take the plan. She ended up driving an hour to see a new one. After a dispute with the insurer about how to count deductibles, leaving her with a $457 pediatrician's bill, she chose a new policy.*[6]

4. Insurers buying up physician practices

Another recent trend that further disrupts patients' established relationships with their doctors is the move by some insurers to buy up physician practices in their efforts to gain competitive advantage in more markets. As examples in 2012:

- UnitedHealth Group's Optum business acquired Monarch Healthcare, an independent practice association based in Irvine, California,
- WellPoint bought CareMore Health Plan, a Medicare Advantage plan in California, Arizona and Nevada with 28 neighborhood care centers, and
- Humana announced its purchase of SeniorBridge Family Cos., an in-home chronic care manager with 1,500 providers; Humana had previously purchased Concentra, which operates urgent- and occupational-care clinics.[7]

5. *Physician burnout and early retirements*

As the health care landscape rapidly changes in the new ACA environment, hospital systems, insurers, and physician groups are the main players. Hospital systems get bigger and buy up more physician practices. Insurers seek larger markets by narrowing their networks with lower-cost doctors. The private practice of medicine is almost gone as more than 60 percent of U.S. physicians are employed by others, usually hospital systems. As a result of this process, physicians have lost clinical autonomy, and have decreasing clout in contract negotiations.

It is therefore not surprising that a large and growing number of U.S. physicians are feeling burned out and are contemplating early retirement. The 2015 Medscape Physician Lifestyle Report found that 46 percent of respondents to a large national study felt that they had burnout, generally defined as loss of enthusiasm for work, a low sense of personal accomplishment, and feelings of cynicism. The highest burnout rates were in critical care (53 percent) and emergency medicine (52 percent), together with one-half of all family physicians, internists, and general surgeons. Burnout rates for family physicians and general internists increased from 43 percent to 50 percent between 2013 and 2015. "Two many bureaucratic tasks" were ranked far as the most common reason for their burnout. Another common reason given was the "increasing computerization of practice," which decreased their face-to-face time with patients.[8] Another recent joint study by the American Medical Association and RAND Corp. found that practice satisfaction is eroding as physicians spend more time on grueling administrative rules, regulations, and paperwork than caring for patients.[9]

According to a 2015 survey by the Deloitte Center for Health Solutions, 62 percent of more than 600 surveyed physicians said that many of their colleagues will retire earlier than planned in the next one to three years. Dissatisfaction, especially in primary care, was attributed to less time with patients, long hours, and dealing with the burdens of Medicare, Medicaid and other regulations.[10]

Summary

As we see from the above, keeping your doctor in this new environment has become very difficult, and for many, impossible—another empty promise of the ACA. We are not just talking about our primary care physicians, but also about the various other specialists we may have been seeing, especially for patients with chronic illness. The new norm is volatility and loss of continuity of care, both of which put the quality of our care at risk. And the costs rapidly escalate for patients with out-of-network physicians, often despite their efforts to try to understand who is in their network.

All of this will get worse as hospital systems and insurers expand and consolidate, as we will discuss in Chapter 14. There is a fix, as we will consider in the last chapter—single-payer national health insurance, which assures full access to doctors and hospitals of our choice anywhere in the country. But meanwhile, let's move to the next chapter to see what challenges patients face if they have to find another doctor.

References:

1. Drobnic Holan, A. "Lie of the year: If you like your doctor, you will be able to keep your doctor." Htpp://www.politifact.com/truth-o-meter/article/2013/dec/12/lie-of-the-year-if-you-like-your-health-plan-keep-it/. PolitiFact.com
2. Beck, M. United Health culls doctors from plan. *Wall Street Journal*, November 16, 2013: B1.
3. Brown, T. Out of network, out of luck. *New York Times*, October 15, 2013.
4. Rosenthal, E. Insured but not covered. *New York Times*, February 8, 2015.
5. Ibid # 4.
6. Ibid # 4.
7. Vesely, R. Marriage of convenience. As they adapt to reform, insurers court historic adversaries: physician practices. *Modern Healthcare*, January 2, 2012.
8. Peckham, C. Physician burnout: it just keeps getting worse. *Medscape*, January 26, 2015.
9. American Medical Association. AMA launches *STEPS Forward* to address physician burnout. June 8, 2015.
10. Pittman, D. Survey: more docs plan to retire early. Practice Management. *MedPage Today*, March 21, 2013.

CHAPTER 9

I HAVE INSURANCE,
BUT CAN'T FIND A DOCTOR

As we have seen in earlier chapters, our health care system is in turmoil. Well intended "reforms" of the ACA have not helped much, and in many cases have increased the turmoil. Even though some 16 million people have gained one or another kind of coverage through the ACA's exchanges or expanded Medicaid, an insurance card does not assure access to care.

Here we look at some of the main reasons that insured patients still have trouble finding doctors after losing them. These are three barriers, all inter-related, posing obstacles to patients finding physicians who will accept their insurance.

Three Main Barriers to Finding a Doctor

1. The primary care shortage

There is a national shortage of about 45,000 primary care physicians. Since no more than 20 percent of U.S. physicians practice primary care, this is a serious problem for millions of newly insured under the ACA gaining access to care. This problem is even more critical in rural areas around the country. In spite of a temporary, two-year raise in primary care reimbursement, many primary care physicians will not accept Medicaid patients because of continuing low reimbursement rates. A recent study of 1,800 physicians listed by private Medicaid plans in 32 states found that one-half would not accept new Medicaid patients or were unavailable at their last known address.[1]

69

There is no shortage in the total number of physicians over-all in the U.S., with a surplus in many non-primary care special-ties.[2] But primary care capacity is limited by ongoing specialty and geographic maldistribution of physicians, due in large part to the higher reimbursement of procedural and non-primary care services. That has led to shortages in primary care, psychiatry, and geriatrics, all more time-intensive specialties.

Here is a typical patient's experience with this problem:

> *Shawn Smith of Seymour, Indiana, newly insured with a subsidized silver-level ACA health plan, spent five months to find a primary care physician on the network who would accept her as a patient. As she said about her search, "I definitely feel like a bad person who is leeching off the system when I call the doctors' offices."*[3]

2. Narrow networks

Two-thirds of health plans offered on the ACA's exchanges across the country offer fewer hospitals and physicians than either pre-ACA employer-sponsored group plans or individual market plans. A 2014 national survey by the Commonwealth Fund of people who had purchased new plans on the exchanges found that 54 percent of respondents reported that their new plan had "all or some" of the doctors they wanted; 39 percent didn't know which doctors were included in their plans, and 5 percent said the new plans had none of the doctors they wanted.[4] Let's see how this has played out in three parts of the country—southern California, Texas, and New York State— in the lives of real people, not sta-tistics.

Southern California

Blue Shield and Anthem Blue Cross, with the two biggest Covered California market shares, each about 30 percent in 2014, have both narrowed their networks. According to Blue Shield, it had 40 percent fewer physicians and 25 percent fewer hospitals in its network in 2014, despite a report by Covered California that it had gained more than 255,000 new enrollees in the open-enrollment period ending early in that year. In its contracts with hospitals and physicians, Blue Shield cut its rates by about 30 percent, defending its cuts as an effort to keep premiums affordable.

Here are two typical patients' experiences with Blue Shield's narrow network:

Noam Friedlander, 40, had health insurance through Covered California, the ACA's exchange in California. With her Blue Shield plan, she hoped to be able to afford surgery for her severely herniated disc. But she found it next to impossible to find a surgeon and hospital in her plan's network that would accept her insurance, even after contacting 20 surgeons and five hospitals. She finally found a hospital that was included in her plan's network, plus a surgeon who operated there but who did not accept her insurance. In the end, she had the surgery but had to take out two credit cards so that she could pay the $16,000 surgeon's bill out-of-pocket.[5]

Ruth Iorio, 35-year-old new mother from Los Angeles, signed up for Blue Cross through Covered California because she found that the plan listed her hospital, UCLA, as accepting that plan. However, after having her baby there in December, she was told that her obstetrician was not on her plan, so she had to pay out-of-pocket. Then she found that her son needs a surgical procedure. After calling more than a dozen doctors covered by her insurance, she was unable to find a doctor willing to do the procedure. As Ruth said about her predicament, 'My insurance is pretty useless. And I'm not fussy about what doctor I see. I don't know what to do. I may drop it just for myself and keep my son on it. It's really depressing. . . . I'm paying $500 a month and every doctor I'm calling is saying, "No, I can't see you." '[6]

When asked about this situation, David Fear, an insurance agent in Sacramento, estimated that about two-thirds of Blue Cross and Blue Shield's specialists had opted out of their networks at that time, two months after the second open-enrollment period ended in April 2014, because of the low reimbursements being offered.[7]

Here is one couple's story about their difficulties in finding doctors in rural areas, where there is usually less choice among insurers (in this case, just two):

> *Christine Ahern and Steve Best of Los Osos in San Luis Obispo County, California had been uninsured for four years after Steve closed down his air conditioning business during the recession. Christine works part-time in a book-store. They purchased coverage through Covered California in 2014, together with about 1.4 million Californians and more than 12,000 other residents of the county, 90 percent of whom qualified for ACA subsidies. Steve was suffering from constant pain from spinal stenosis, and hoped that their new coverage would allow him to receive treatment. But they soon found that his primary care doctor's medical group would not accept Covered California insurance. Nor would the urgent care center, the pain management center, or the orthopedic surgery group he went to for consultation. Fortunately, however, they found a general practitioner who would accept him for care, who even found him a neurosurgeon who would treat him for his spinal stenosis. As Christine said, 'For the most part, we're pleased with Covered California, but the biggest problem is finding doctors, especially specialists.'* [8]

Texas

Even when patients are fortunate enough to find a primary care physician, it is frequently even more difficult for them to gain access to non-primary care specialists.

Dr. Charu Sawhney is a primary care physician at the Hope Clinica federally qualified health center in southwest Houston. Many of her patients are uninsured immigrants from Asia. Some have purchased health plans on the exchanges, and Dr. Sawhney has had just as much trouble getting them specialist care as the uninsured. She was able to get an oncologist, Dr. Paul Zhang, to see one of her patients, who had a Blue Cross Blue Shield silver HMO plan, but their joint efforts to find a surgeon were unsuccessful. The two largest hospital chains in Houston, Houston Methodist and Memorial Hermann, are not in the plan's network, nor is Houston's premier cancer hospital, MD Anderson Cancer Center. They finally found a surgeon to accept his care, but not one specializing in cancer surgery, and the patient's cancer had already spread to 30 lymph nodes. Dr. Sawhney worries that her insured patients will decide that the cost of insurance isn't worth it.[9]

Concerning the chronic problem that primary care physicians have in getting their patients specialist care, Dr. Elizabeth Torres, a general internist in the Houston suburb of Sugar Land and president of the Harris County Medical Society, fears that there may be a backlash among primary care physicians, not because the narrow network HMOs have lower reimbursements, but because it's too difficult to find specialists. As she says,

'There is no guarantee that if you see the [specialist's] name on the website, that they're actually participating, and that's an issue. . . If it's going to cost us a lot of hassle administratively as far as finding the specialists, then it's going to be less likely and less favorable for us to actually want to be part of the plan.'[10]

New York State

Finding a specialist for patients insured through the exchanges is also a big problem in New York State, as this patient's story illustrates:

> *Jon Fougner, a recent graduate of Yale Law School, called 30 doctors after getting his new ACA exchange plan. Among those 30, they either weren't taking new patients, weren't in the plan, didn't return calls, or their contact information was incorrect. He sued Empire Blue Cross for his inability to find a physician in the plan.*[11]

Dr. Andrew Kleinman, a plastic surgeon and president of the Medical Society of the State of New York, tells us that his members complain that rates in exchange plans can be 50 percent lower than those in commercial plans, and that some doctors are limiting the numbers of new patients they take with these policies, if they take them at all. As he says:

> *The exchanges have become much like Medicaid. . . . Physicians who are in solo practices have to be careful to not take too many patients reimbursed at lower rates or they're not going to be in business very long.'*[12]

Is it any better for Medicaid and Medicare patients?

Unfortunately, the problem of private insurers dropping physicians from their networks, with little notice and no appeal, also is common in both primary care and the other specialties. In Tennessee, as an example, Medicaid patients in UnitedHealthcare's Community Plan received a letter in 2014 stating that their primary care physicians would no longer be included in the plan's network. In the previous year, thousands of physicians in many specialties were similarly dropped from private Medicare Advantage plans, without reasons being given, in states including Connecticut, Rhode Island, Florida and Ohio. Insurers, of course, defend their actions as leading to greater efficiency and long-term cost savings, both claims unproven. In response to this problem, the American Academy of Family Physicians' Board Chair, Dr. Jeffrey Cain, sent a letter to UnitedHealthcare stating:

The so-called 'network optimization' is disruptive to patients and their physicians and, in our opinion, a violation of the core tenets of quality primary care. . . . If patients go to a new physician, they lose the trusting relationship established with their physician. The value of those physicians rests on their familiarity and unique experiences with each of their patients to create and manage an appropriate treatment plan.' [13]

Is there any fix for these narrowed networks?

Federal guidance for the adequacy of insurance networks under the ACA are so general as to not be very helpful—marketplace plans must maintain "a network that is sufficient in number and types of providers" so that "all services will be accessible without

FIGURE 9.1

STATES WITH MARKETPLACE PLANS SUBJECT TO ONE OR MORE QUANTITATIVE STANDARDS FOR NETWORK ADEQUACY, JANUARY 2014

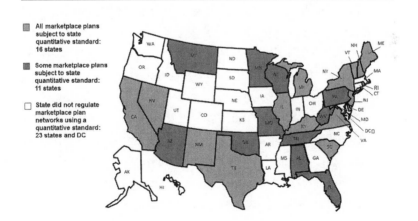

All marketplace plans subject to state quantitative standard: 16 states

Some marketplace plans subject to state quantitative standard: 11 states

State did not regulate marketplace plan networks using a quantitative standard: 23 states and DC

Notes: State network adequacy standards may apply broadly, to all network plans, or more narrowly, to specified network designs (e.g., HMOs) or plan types (e.g., marketplace plans).

Sources: Authors' analysis Issue Brief. Implementing the Affordable Care Act state regulation of marketplace plan provider networks. *The Commonwealth Fund*, May 5, 2015. Reprinted with permission.

reasonable delay." Oversight and regulation of networks are left to the states, some of which impose requirements on such matters as availability of primary care physicians in terms of numbers and distance, maximal waiting times, minimal ratios of providers to enrollees, and updating of provider directories. But as Figure 9.1 shows, regulation by states was loose and highly variable in 2014.[14]

3. Long wait times

When one is fortunate enough to find a new doctor, the next step is how long the wait will be before the first appointment. Here again, waiting times vary widely across the country by specialty, type of visit, market, and socio-economic factors. In our largely for-profit market-based system, *if* one's insurance is accepted, wait times for such procedures as a hip replacement, an MRI, or a Botox injection can be relatively short. But wait times for less reimbursed, time-consuming office visits, especially in primary care, geriatrics and psychiatry, are much longer.

A study by Merritt Hawkins, a physician staffing firm, polled some 1,400 medical offices in 15 large metropolitan areas across the country in 2013. It found that long wait times for non-emergency care are still common, as they were before the ACA. As examples, the national average wait time to see a dermatologist for a skin examination was 29 days, 32 days to see a cardiologist in Washington, and 66 days to schedule a physician examination in Boston (despite being the city having the most doctors per capita, mostly specialists).[15] As a result of these long wait times, patients are forced to seek care in emergency rooms or urgent care centers more frequently, in both cases without continuity of care, and often with difficulties arranging ongoing necessary care. Figure 9.2 shows how poorly access to primary care is in the U.S. when compared to 10 other advanced countries.[16]

FIGURE 9.2

ACCESS TO AFTER-HOURS CARE

Primary care physicians, 2012
Practice has arrangement for patients'
after-hours care to see doctor or nurse

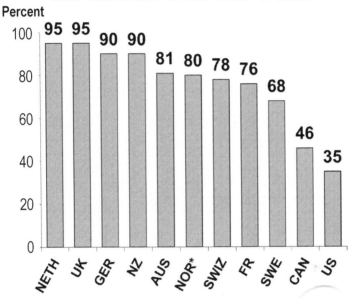

Source: Osborn, R, Schoen, C. 2013 International Health Policy Survey in Eleven Countries. *The Commonwealth Fund,* November 2013. Reprinted with permission.

Summary

In the overall picture, a battle rages on between the three main players—hospitals, insurers, and physician groups—in the competition for expanded markets under the ACA. The battle, of course, is all about money. Insurers want to narrow their networks and contract with lower-cost hospitals and physician groups. Hospitals want to increase their market power, and charge what they can. Both have considerable latitude to set their rates. Physicians, mostly employed today by hospitals, are caught in the middle with less negotiating power. They often refuse care to patients on the basis of unacceptably low reimbursement rates imposed by private insurers or Medicaid, thereby distorting ever-changing networks.

So we have to conclude that an insurance card doesn't mean access to care, despite the promises of the ACA, and that lower-premium plans have more restricted networks that put patients at a disadvantage. In the next chapter, we will consider just how much coverage goes with health insurance these days.

References:

1. Pear, R. Half of doctors listed as serving Medicaid patients are unavailable, investigation finds. *New York Times*, December 8, 2014.
2. Makaroff, LA, Green, LA, Petterson, SM et al. Trends in physician's supply and population growth. *Amer Fam Phys* 87 (7), April 2013.
3. O'Donnell, JO. Some doctors wary of taking insurance exchange patients. *USA Today*, October 28, 2014.
4. Feibel, C. Specialty care is a challenge in some ACA plans. *Houston Public Media, NPR* and *Kaiser Health News*, July 16, 2014.
5. Ibid # 3.
6. Miles, K. How Obamacare leaves some people without doctors. *Huffington Post,* April 10, 2014.
7. Ibid # 6.
8. Ibid # 6.
9. Lavelle, J. Finding doctors who take Covered California plans isn't easy, locals say. *The Tribune News*, May 29, 2014.
10. Ibid #4.
11. Ibid #3
12. Ibid #3, quoting Kleinman, A
13. Laff, M. AAFP denounces 'arbitrary elimination' of physicians from insurers' networks. *AAFP News*, July 29, 2014.
14. Issue Brief. Implementing the Affordable Care Act state regulation of marketplace plan provider networks. *The Commonwealth Fund*, May 5, 2015.
15. Rosenthal, E. The health care waiting game. *New York Times*, July 5, 2014.
16. Osborn, R, Schoen, C. 2013 International Health Policy Survey in Eleven Countries. *The Commonwealth Fund*, November 2013.

CHAPTER 10

I HAVE INSURANCE,
BUT ITS COVERAGE IS POOR

Private health insurers are cashing in on expanded subsidized markets of the ACA by attracting enrollees with lower premiums, adding higher deductibles and other cost sharing, and minimizing their own exposure to health care costs that are increasingly shouldered by patients and their families. Although they can no longer deny coverage based on pre-existing conditions and have to meet other requirement of the ACA in marketing their policies, they still try to avoid sicker patients if they can and have many ways to extract more profits in doing so.

Here are some of the main ways that they can add to their own financial bottom lines and keep investors on Wall Street happy.

How Private Insurers Game the ACA for More Profits

1. The metal plans

The ACA established four levels of coverage for health insurers—the so-called "metals"—with actuarial values (what insurers pay vs. what patients pay) ranging from 60 percent (bronze) and 70 percent (silver) to 80 percent (gold) and 90 percent (platinum). Silver plans have been the most popular on the exchanges, leaving patients with 30 percent of their health care costs, plus the cost sharing that was required to get and maintain their policies. The lower the actuarial value of the plan, the higher the deductible. One-half of bronze plans in seven large U.S. cities require enrollees to pay the deductible (often $5,000) before covering a doctor's visit.[1] Not content with these relatively low actuarial values, America's Health Insurance Plans (AHIP), the industry's trade group, has been lobbying (so far unsuccessfully) for an even poorer metal plan—a "copper" plan, with only 50 percent actuarial value.[2]

2. Wide marketing of high-deductible plans

We all know that deductibles have been rising all the time, for example, with a 42 percent increase in 2013 to an *average* of $5,081 a year in 2014.[3] Here are two typical stories of the difficult trade-off between premium affordability and out-of-pocket exposure through high-deductibles:

> *Edward Frank, in his 50s and looking for a job in Reynoldsville, Pennsylvania, bought a plan in late 2013 with a $6,000 deductible through the federal exchange. He could not afford a plan with a lower deductible at the time. He had to pay $4,000 out of his own pocket when he needed treatment for shoulder pain. As he said, 'Unless you get desperately ill and in the hospital for weeks, it's going to cost you more to have this plan and pay the premiums than to pay the bill just outright. . . . The deductibles are so high, you don't get much of anything out of it.*[4]

> *Mike Tilbury, 62, retired from the pharmaceutical industry in New Orleans, bought an individual plan for his 26-year-old son, Patrick, whose previous health insurance had cost $130 a month with a $1,300 deductible. That policy did not meet the ACA's requirements. The new policy, without eligibility for subsidies, cost $212 a month with a $6,000 annual deductible. As Mr. Tilbury said, 'That puts us in a real tough spot if anything happens to him. His deductible increased by six times, so how is the model working? He'll most likely never get much benefit from this unless he becomes seriously ill or injured.'*[5]

3. Narrow networks

As we saw in the last chapter, insurers are narrowing their networks, focusing on lower-cost physicians and hospitals, in an effort to keep their premiums attractive to more enrollees. Narrow networks serve the financial interests of insurers, but don't serve patients well through restricted choice of hospitals and physicians, disruption of continuity of care, and increased out-of-pocket costs when they have to see out-of-network providers.

A recent analysis of almost 400 physician networks in silver-level plans sold across the country in 2014 showed the extreme extent to which networks have shrunk. Almost one-third of these networks were small, covering only 10 to 25 percent of physicians in a plan's region, while 11 percent were "extra small", including less than 10 percent of physicians.[6]

Even when patients are careful and fortunate enough to be in networks that include most of the hospitals and physicians of their choice, they may still be blind-sided by unexpected out-of-network costs, as we saw in Chapter 2.

Another unwelcome surprise for many patients is when they go to an emergency room at a hospital within their plan's network only to find that the E. R. physicians are out-of-network. This is quite common, since two-thirds of U.S. hospitals contract out emergency care. Some emergency medicine staffing groups, many of which service a large number of hospitals nationally or locally, opt out of all insurance plans. In most states, physicians can bill patients for the difference between their charges and what insurers pay. In Texas, where UnitedHealthcare, Humana, and Blue Cross-Blue Shield are the biggest insurers, up to one-half of participating hospitals have no in-network emergency physicians.[7]

4. Offering other plans not meeting ACA requirements

The ACA gave employers a way to get around its requirements for ESI plans by allowing them to offer plans that fall short of these requirements if they offer one plan than does. Another way that insurers can evade these rules is to market short-term plans that last less than 12 months.[8]

5. Specialty drug tiers

As the costs of specialty drugs—the very expensive drugs used for such conditions as cancer, rheumatoid arthritis, multiple sclerosis and hepatitis C—continue to soar, insurers are charging enrollees a set percentage of the costs of the drugs as coinsurance. The lower the actuarial value of the plan, of course, the higher the coinsurance. At first, co\insurance requirement of 30 percent were common, but now they are rising, as shown in Table 10.1, and becoming unaffordable for many sick patients.[9] What that means for cancer patients with the most popular silver plans, who need a chemotherapy drug costing $100,000 a year, is annual costs of more than $30,000 for that drug.

6. Narrow definitions of "medical necessity"

Mental health care has long been an issue in this country in its being accorded lower priority than physical illness. For many years, insurers and employers have imposed more limits on treatment of mental health conditions than for treatment of physical conditions. Compared to physical conditions, insurance coverage for mental health care has typically included higher cost-sharing, more restrictive limits on the number of inpatient days and outpatient visits, different pre-authorization requirements, and separate annual and lifetime caps on coverage.

In response to this problem, Congress passed the Mental Health Parity Act in 1996, championed by Senators Paul Wellstone (D-MN) and Pete Domenici (R-NM). That law prohibited large employer-sponsored group health plans from imposing higher annual or lifetime dollar limits on mental health benefits than those for medical or surgical benefits. Although an important beginning, the law did not address treatment limits, differences in cost shar-

TABLE 10.1

PERCENT OF EXCHANGE PLANS WITH COINSURANCE ABOVE 30 PERCENT FOR SPECIALTY TIER DRUGS

Bronze (60 % actuarial value)
2014	38%
2015	52%

Silver (70 % actuarial value)
2014	27%
2015	41%

Gold (80 % actuarial value)
2014	20%
2015	22%

Platinum (90 % actuarial value)
2014	17%
2015	26%

ing, and limits on mental health coverage in managed care plans. In further response, Congress passed the Mental Health Parity and Addiction Equity Act of 2008, which requires group health plans and insurers to ensure that cost sharing and treatment limitations are no more restrictive for mental health or substance abuse disorders than those for medical and surgical benefits. Parity is also required for aggregate lifetime and annual dollar limits.[10]

The following patient's story, however, illustrates how far we still are from mental health parity:

Michael Kamins, a marketing professor at the State University of New York, Stony Brook, was enraged when he opened a letter from his health insurer to find that it was no longer necessary for his 20-year-old son with bipolar disorder to see his psychiatrist twice a week. His son had recently been hospitalized twice and rescued from the brink of suicide, but the insurer would now pay for just two visits per month. His son later became violent and suicidal, and was re-hospitalized eight months later. His father is suing the insurer, OptumHealth Behavioral Solutions, which denies that it left the patient with insufficient care. Michael has also contracted with another insurer, which provided better coverage, and allowed his son to stabilize and return to college.[11]

The National Alliance on Mental Illness, an advocacy group for people with mental illness and their families, has recently reported that patients are denied payment for treatment on the basis of "not being medically necessary" twice as often for mental health conditions as for physical conditions. Enforcement of mental health parity provisions are still lax, more litigation is brewing, and insurers have been slow to release documents concerning alleged parity violations.[12]

7. Other fine print provisions

Many restrictions in coverage hide in the fine print of many health insurance policies. "Illegal activity" is one such little-known example that is frequently used by insurers to deny coverage for patients injured in various contexts ranging from traffic infractions to gun accidents. Here is one example of this practice, which Crystal Patterson, an attorney in Minneapolis and chairwoman of the American Bar Association's committee on fiduciary litigations, tells us is "more common than people think."

Monroe Bird III, 21, was sitting in a car with a friend one night in the parking lot of an apartment house complex in Tulsa, Oklahoma, when he was apprehended by a security guard. The guard had been instructed to watch for couples having sex in that parking lot. There was no video of the ensuing encounter that involved the guard drawing his gun and shooting Monroe, leaving him paralyzed from the neck down. Although he was not charged or convicted of any crime, the insurer denied coverage on the basis of "illegal activity." Without insurance, the family could not move him to a rehabilitation center specializing in spinal cord injuries. One month after discharge from the hospital, he died at home of a preventable complication.[13]

Underinsurance in America: A Growing Epidemic

Despite some progress under the ACA, we are seeing a growing epidemic of *underinsurance* in this country, whether through employers, the exchanges, or Medicaid. A 2014 report from the Kaiser Family Foundation estimates that one in three Americans have difficulty in paying their medical bills, even when insured. It lists these ways that insured people may be forced into burdensome medical debt:

- "In-network cost-sharing
- Out-of-network care
- Health plan coverage limits or exclusions
- Unaffordable premiums
- Other factors unrelated to insurance, such as income loss due to illness"

The report also notes these ways that the ACA does not address the underlying causes of medical debt:

- "High cost-sharing will persist under many plans.
- Limited protections for out-of-network care
- Limits on essential health benefits standards
- Lack of resources for consumer assistance."[14]

The following two markers suggest the prevalence and consequences of underinsurance:

- Almost one-third of low-income families (0-125 percent of FPL) spend more than 5 percent of their meager incomes on medical expenses, while many forgo or delay necessary care or medications because of costs.[15]
- Many states have narrowed provider networks and reduced Medicaid coverage[16]

Trudy Lieberman, long experienced journalist with a focus on health care and author of *Slanting the Story: The Forces that Shape the News*, sums up the impact of the ACA in these words:

> *It's bad enough that the ACA is fattening up the health-care industry and hollowing out coverage for the middle class. Even worse, the law is accelerating what I call the Great Cost Shift, which transfers the growing price of medical care to patients themselves through high-deductibles, coinsurance (the patient's share of the cost for a specific service, calculated as a percentage), copayments (a set fee paid for a specific service), and limited provider networks (which sometimes offer so little choice that patients end up seeking out-of-network care and paying on their own). What was once good, comprehensive insurance for a sizable number of Americans is being reduced to coverage for only the most serious, and most expensive, of illnesses.[17]*

Summary

As we have seen in this and earlier chapters, in spite of the ACA, a large part of our population is having to deal with rising premium costs for insurance of less and less value, more cost-sharing, and restricted choices of hospitals and physicians. We can expect these pressures to come together in a growing public backlash that will force us to look at the three options to be discussed in Part Three of this book.

References:

1. Appleby, J. Consumers beware: not all health plans cover a doctor's visit before the deductible is met. *Kaiser Health News*, December 23, 2013.
2. Andrews, M. Proposal to add skimpier "copper" plans to marketplace raises concerns. *Kaiser Health News*, July 1, 2014.
3. Scism. L, Martin, TW. Deductibles fuel new worries of health-law sticker shock. *Wall Street Journal*, December 9, 2013.
4. *Associated Press*. Health care insecurity. Poll: many insured struggle with medical bills, October 13, 2014.
5. Armour, S. Health costs hinge on Supreme Court ruling. *Wall Street Journal*, May 26, 2015.
6. Andrews, M. Study finds almost half of health law plans offer very limited physician networks. *Kaiser Health News*, June 26, 2015.
7. Rosenthal, E. Costs can go up fast when E. R. is in network but the doctors are not. *New York Times,* September 28, 2014.
8. Andrews, M. Short-term plans can skirt health law requirements. *Kaiser Health News*, October 28, 2013.
9. Pearson, CF. Exchange plans increase costs of specialty drugs for 2015. *Avalere*, December 2, 2014.
10. Goodell, S. Mental health parity. Health Policy Brief. *Health Affairs*, April 3, 2014.
11. Gold, J. Advocates say mental health 'parity' law is not fulfilling its promise. *Kaiser Health News*, August 3, 2015.
12. Ibid # 11.
13. Rabin, RC. 'Illegal activity' fine print leaves some insured, but uncovered. *New York Times*, July 20, 2015.
14. Pollitz, K, Cox, C, Lucia, K et al. Medical debt among people with health insurance. *Kaiser Family Foundation*, January 2014.
15. Magge, H, Cabral, HJ, Kazis, LE et al. Prevalence and predictors of underinsurance among low-income adults. *J Gen Intern Med* 2013. doi: 10.1007/s11606-013-2354-z
16. Galewitz, P, Fleming, M. 13 states aim to limit Medicaid. *USA Today*, July 24, 2012.
17. Lieberman, T. Wrong prescription? The failed promise of the Affordable Care Act. *Harper's Magazine*, July 2015.

CHAPTER 11

I HAVE INSURANCE,
BUT CAN'T AFFORD CARE

The ACA has brought some protections to patients in an effort to make health care more affordable. These include subsidies/ tax credits for many millions of people helping to make insurance more affordable, especially for people with incomes at or below 200 percent of the FPL who purchase their plans on state or federal exchanges. The ACA has also introduced annual and lifetime caps on maximum out-of-pocket spending for health care (MOOP). But remarkably lacking is any significant way to rein in health care prices, be it for insurance, hospitals, drugs, medical devices, or other health care costs. Here we examine the shortfalls of the ACA as real patients try to navigate this new system even as they are armed with a new insurance card.

Some Ways that the Newly Insured Still Can't Afford Health Care

1. Can't meet deductible

Insurers have put their emphasis on keeping premiums competitive to attract more enrollees, but lower premiums mean higher cost-sharing, especially for deductibles, which go up all the time. A 2014 survey by the Kaiser Family Foundation found that average deductibles for bronze plans purchased on the exchange were $5,051 for individuals and $10,386 for families; averages for silver plans were $2,907 and $6,078, respectively.¹ Here is one patient's experience with high-deductibles, unfortunately all too common.

> *Patricia Wanderlich, 61, had a brain hemorrhage in 2011, and spent weeks in a hospital intensive care unit. She has a second, smaller aneurism, that needs monitoring. She works part-time for a landscaping company outside Chicago. She purchased a new plan through an ACA exchange with a $6,000 annual deductible. She is skipping this year's brain scan, hoping for the best, because of this high-deductible. As she says, To spend thousands of dollars just making sure it hasn't grown? I don't have that money. At the next open-enrollment period, she was planning to switch to a plan with a narrower network of doctors, even at the cost of losing continuity with her specialists. As she said, 'At this point, I am resigned. . . . A $6,000 deductible—that's just staggering. I never thought I'd say this, but how many minutes until I get Medicare?'*²

2. Out-of-network care doesn't count toward your insurance deductible.

One might assume that the ACA's cap on out-of-pocket health care spending would cover across the board, but that is not true, as this patient found:

> *Dr. Rebecca Love of Moab, Utah, has degenerative arthritis and other medical problems. She was paying $422 a month for a plan with a deductible of $6,000. She paid more than $6,000 in medical bills in 2014, but that didn't count toward her deductible, since her care was in Grand Junction, Colorado, more than 100 miles away. She would have had to travel to Salt Lake City, much farther away over a treacherous mountain pass, to see specialists in her own network. As she said, 'Medical care costs too much and health insurance as it stands doesn't address this. What have we become?'*³

3. Forgo care because of high-deductible

Delaying or forgoing care has become all too common. A 2014 Gallup poll found that one in three Americans said that they or a family member delayed medical care because of cost in that year. Here is one example, among many, showing how sensitive patients have become to health care costs:

> *Jessica and Doyle Lewis have a family plan with a $6,000 deductible. She is a project manager at Wells Fargo & Co. When their son was born, they knew that he would be an only child, but deferred a vasectomy and other medical care because of the high deductible.*[4]

A recent study sheds light on how pervasive this increased sensitivity to health care costs has become. Researchers looked at one large company providing ESI before and after the company shifted almost all of its employees and dependents—more than 150,000—from an insurance plan providing first-dollar coverage without cost-sharing to a high-deductible plan covering 78 percent of medical spending on average. Their findings showed that increased cost-sharing leads to less medical spending:

- Cuts in medical spending were across the board, including preventive services, imaging procedures, outpatient and in-patient hospital services, emergency room care, and drug purchases.
- Patients did not price-shop after the switch, or move to lower-cost providers.
- Even the sickest 25 percent, based on prior diagnoses each year, reduced their spending by one-quarter after the shift.[5]

There are other recent examples of how frequently health care is being delayed or avoided. A recent Gallup poll found that as many as 16 million adults with chronic conditions have avoided seeing doctors because of out-of-pocket costs.[6] Cancer patients typically face out-of-pocket expenses for their treatment as high as one-half of their average annual household income.[7] Despite having insurance, many are forced to reduce the frequency of their prescribed medications or cut their spending on food and clothing in order to make ends meet.[8]

4. Can't make copayment

Mark Yuschak, 57, of Jackson, New Jersey, had a silver plan with a deductible of $3,000. When his wife had a digestive disorder and went to a nearby emergency room, they presented their insurance card and filled out all the forms. But they were soon told, 'You don't have a copayment, you're free to go.' Later, they received a bill for more than $1,000, but their insurance would not cover it because they had not met their deductible.[9]

5. Unaffordable coinsurance

Sarah Truman has a well-paying job in Portland, Oregon, and has health insurance through an ACA exchange. She takes an intravenous drug, much like chemotherapy, for her psoriatic arthritis. She has to pay a 20 percent coinsurance for this drug, $3,000 for a $15,000 a month drug. She is still able to work, but has to go to food banks to afford her children's food.[10]

This appears to be an example of "adverse tiering", whereby insurers put some drugs into such high tiers that high coinsurance requirements will discourage sicker patients from enrolling in their plans. As one example, the AIDS Institute has found that some Florida insurers put all HIV medications into the highest tier, including generics. The Department of Health and Human Services (HHS) is reviewing whether this kind of drug pricing discriminates against people based on pre-existing conditions, and may soon issue a ruling on this subject.[11]

6. Maximal out-of-pocket spending for health care (MOOP) caps with inadequate protection

The ACA has helped to prevent insurmountable medical bills by setting $6,600 per-person, per-year cap on out-of-pocket costs for individuals and $13,200 for families. But for many people confronting very large medical bills, this is inadequate protection, as illustrated by this family's experience:

Christian and Jaycee Garcia of Silver Spring, Maryland, have been hard hit by medical bills for care of their 20-month-old son, CJ, born with the rare genetic disorder prune-belly syndrome (Eagle Barrett Syndrome) and severe scoliosis. He has already had twelve surgeries and faces more to rebuild his digestive system and urinary tract and to insert metal rods next to his spine so that he can sit up without a brace. Although Christian earns $60,000 a year as a restaurant manager, monthly expenses, including payments on medical bills account for all of his take-home pay of about $3,000 a month. The family is paying more than $700 a month in premiums for his work plan and another privately purchased plan for his wife and children. They have been forced to sell their wedding rings and move into Christian's stepfather's home, where they pay $500 in monthly rent. They explored the possibility of Social Security Income to help with their son's disability, but were told that, because of their income, they would have to have two more children to become eligible. As Christian said, 'You have to be really at a point where you can't live and can't help yourself anymore. We're trying to do everything the right way, and help cannot be given.'[12]

7. MOOP maximum applies only in network

Dennis Doman, 64, a former warehouse manager in the Philadelphia, Pennsylvania area, had a UnitedHealth-

93

care Silver Compass 100 plan when he had sudden onset of bleeding through his mouth. He called 911 and was hospitalized at a nearby hospital with a presumptive diagnosis of a gastrointestinal problem. He was sent the next day to Thomas Jefferson University Hospital, where he was found to have a cancerous mass in his neck. After many subsequent surgeries and emergency room visits, his medical bills grew to almost $200,000. Although he thought his insurance would cover these bills, and although his physicians also thought so, he soon discovered that his insurance excluded out-of-network care. Although every health insurance plan allows you to go to the nearest hospital in an emergency, once you are stabilized, you must transfer to an in-network doctor or hospital for your insurance to cover. Otherwise, one is responsible for the full cost of care, and the ACA's yearly maximum of out-of-pocket costs will not apply.[13]

This experience, unfortunately, is not at all uncommon. Unanticipated out-of-network costs blindside many patients who thought their insurance would cover them.

8. Drug prices unaffordable

Sandra Grooms, 52, has health insurance through her job as a general manager at a janitorial supply company in Augusta, Georgia. While undergoing chemotherapy for metastatic breast cancer, she was advised by her oncologist to take a drug that was covered by her insurance but required a 20 percent copayment—$976 for each 14-day supply of the two pills. She could not afford these copayments, and opted instead for an intravenous drug with a lower copay of $100 a month. As she said, 'Requiring huge copayments sharply affects middle class people who are working and trying to make a living, even though they *may be living with a serious illness.'* [14]

The costs of specialty drugs for cancer are going through the roof. New cancer drugs are routinely priced above $100,000 a year, about twice the average annual household income.[15] As they go up, the copayments also increase, today often higher than Sandra experienced. Oncologists are increasingly alarmed that costs of cancer drugs are now beyond reach of many of their patients. And many are aware that the high costs of these drugs has nothing to do with their effectiveness. Dr. Vinay Prasad, chief fellow in oncology at the National Cancer Institute, studied all cancer drugs approved between 2009 and 2013. No difference was found in costs of drugs that improve survival the most and those with no effect on survival. He has this to say:

> *Our ultimate consensus was that there is no rational basis for drug prices. It's not based on how novel they are or how well they work. It's based on what the market will bear.*[16]

Other drugs are also at crisis levels. More than half a million Americans had prescription drug costs over $50,000 a year in 2014, while about 139,000 accounted for more than $100,000, triple that in 2013.[17]

Gilead's new drug, Sovaldi, approved in 2013 for the treatment of Hepatitis C, has become a poster child for exorbitant drug prices. It can cure that disease in 90 percent of patients over a 12-week treatment period, but at a cost of $1,000 a pill or $84,000 per course of treatment. By comparison, costs in Europe for Sovaldi are about $55,000 per treatment and as little as $900 in India.[18] Since Hepatitis C affects some 3 million people in the U.S. and successful treatment can prevent later liver cancer or the need for a liver transplant, Gilead's pricing policies have created a firestorm of protest from payers, policymakers, and leaders in public health. States are especially vulnerable to Sovaldi as a budget breaker. As Jeff Myers, president and CEO of Medicaid Health Plans of America, says:

> *Medicaid programs across the country are sharply restricting access to Sovaldi, offering it only to the sickest patients. If the drug had been priced more rationally, my expectation is that states would try to treat everyone they could get a hold of. Imagine if Jonas Salk, when he invented the polio vaccine, had priced it like Gilead. We'd still have polio.*[19]

Big increases in costs of generic drugs are also a problem, as this patient found:

> *When Carol Ann Riha, 57, a retired journalist in West Des Moines, Iowa, filled her prescription for the cholesterol-lowering drug, Pravastatin, she couldn't believe the price increase. What for months had cost $4 for a 30-day supply had jumped to almost $19. The pharmacist could not explain the difference.*[20]

Summary

Affordability of health care has become a crisis for ordinary Americans as insurers prosper with their expanded markets subsidized by taxpayers. People are paying a lot for inadequate insurance, are losing choice of their doctors and hospitals, and are burdened by growing medical debt, and even bankruptcy, as we will see in the next chapter.

References:

1. Goodnough, A, Pear, R. Unable to meet the deductible. *New York Times*, October 17, 2014.
2. Ibid # 1.
3. Ibid # 1.
4. Armour, S. As consumers pay more, health care delayed. *Wall Street Journal*, December 4, 2014.
5. Handel, B. Health care cost-sharing prompts consumers to make big cuts in medical spending. *The Conversation*, June 15, 2015.
6. The editors. Out of Pocket, out of control. *Bloomberg View*, February 16, 2015.
7. Kantarjian, H, Steensma, D, Sanjuan, JR et al. High cancer drug prices in the United States: reasons and proposed solutions. *Journal of Oncology Practice*, May 6, 2014.
8. Zafarm, SY, Peppercorn, JM, Schrag, D et al. The financial toxicity of cancer treatment: a pilot study assessing out-of-pocket expenses and the insured cancer patient's experience. *Oncologist* 18: 381-390, 2013.
9. Ibid # 1.
10. Fitzsimons, T. Advocates say insurers are driving away sick customers. *Marketplace*, June 11, 2015.
11. Ibid # 10.
12. O'Donnell, MJ, Ungar, L. Obamacare reduces maximum out-of-pocket costs, but not enough for some. *USA Today*, August 3, 2015.
13. Calandra, R. Beware: your insurer may define a health emergency differently than you do. *Philadelphia Inquirer*, June 22, 2015.
14. Appleby, J. Got insurance? You still may pay a steep price for prescriptions. *Kaiser Health News*, October 13, 2014.
15. Szalso, Z. Skyrocketing drug prices leave cures out of reach for some patients. *USA Today*, June 15, 2015.
16. Ibid # 15.
17. Berkrot, B. Number of Americans using $100,000 in medicines triples— Express Scripts. Reuters, May 13, 2015.
18. LaMattina, J. Even at $900 (vs. $84,000 in U.S.) Hep C cure Sovaldi's cost could be unacceptable in India. *Forbes*. August 8, 2014.
19. Ibid # 15.
20. Jaret, P. Prices spike for some generics. *AARP Bulletin*, July-August 2015.

*In a country as wealthy as ours, nobody should go bank-
rupt if they get sick.*

—President Obama, in a press conference
defending the Affordable Care Act[1]

CHAPTER 12

I HAD INSURANCE,
BUT WENT BANKRUPT ANYWAY

*Simon and Marsha Sutherland, residents in the Orlan-
do, Florida area, both have good jobs, she as a full-time
reading teacher and he as manager of a chain pizzeria.
They had a combined income of about $100,000 a year,
as well as two major health insurance policies. But they
were forced into foreclosure and bankruptcy after almost
four years of high medical bills for their daughter Ellie's
care. Shortly after her birth, Ellie appeared to have a sei-
zure, and was transferred to the Winnie Palmer neonatal
intensive care for a 25-day stay, an initial $74,000 bill.
Meanwhile, without a definitive clinical diagnosis, the
bills accumulated as Ellie was nearly deaf, couldn't sit up,
was prone to high fevers, and had other medical problems.
She was hospitalized twice at the Johns Hopkins University Hospital, and she had almost weekly visits to Central
Florida specialists for her hearing, eyes, spine and gastrointestinal problems. Marsha continued to work part-
time until she needed to be home for continuous care of
Ellie. They applied for Social Security disability, but were
turned down, as they were for Medicaid. Even after the
family was down to a single income, they had too much to
qualify for either program. Despite all her treatment, Ellie
died just short of her fourth birthday in 2011.[2]*

With this bankruptcy, the Sutherlands joined some 1.7 million Americans who are bankrupted by medical bills every year, even though three-quarters of them have health insurance. This is a problem of long standing, predating the ACA, as revealed by two large national studies. In 2001, illness and medical bills contributed to about one-half of all personal bankruptcies, involving about 2.2 million debtors and their dependents.[3] A follow-up national study was done in 2007, which found that medical bankruptcies had climbed to 62 percent of all bankruptcies in the U.S. Most of those bankrupted were middle class, owned their own homes, had attended college, and had held responsible jobs. Seventy-eight percent had health insurance when they got sick, mostly private coverage.[4]

The ACA is modeled after the Massachusetts health reform bill, enacted in 2006, requiring people to buy health insurance. While it did cut the number of uninsured from 10.4 to 4.4 percent of the state's population (the lowest of any of the 50 states), the actual number of people filing for medical bankruptcy increased from 7,504 in 2007 to 10,093 in 2009. The reasons for this result are given by the researchers who did the earlier national studies cited above:

> *Health costs in the state have risen sharply since reform was enacted. Even before the changes in health care laws, most medical bankruptcies in Massachusetts—as in other states—afflicted middle-class families with health insurance. High premium costs and gaps in coverage— co-payments, deductibles and uncovered services—often left insured families liable for substantial out-of-pocket costs. None of that changed. . . . Massachusetts' health reform, like the national law modeled after it, takes many of the uninsured and makes them underinsured, typically giving them a skimpy, defective private policy that's like an umbrella that melts in the rain: the protection's not there when you need it.'*[5]

Looking back 40 years shows a steady and unrelenting erosion in the level of protection provided by health insurance. According to the 1977 National Medical Expenditure Survey (NMES), 12.6% of individuals with private coverage had a 1% annual probability of incurring out-of-pocket (OOP) medical expenses more than 10 percent of family income, a good definition of underinsurance.[6] By that definition, underinsurance increased to 18.5 percent of those with private insurance in 1994.[7] More recently, a series of surveys of non-elderly adults by the Commonwealth Fund found that the proportion spending more than 10% of income on OOP costs and premiums rose from 21 % in 2001 to 32% in 2010.[8]

Translating all this down to concrete terms, a hypothetical 56-year old in 2013 with an income of $45,900 (399 percent of the FPL and thus eligible for ACA subsidies) would pay an estimated $4,361 in premiums for an individual bronze plan, and up to $4,167 for additional deductibles and copayments for covered services. With an income of $46,100, (401 percent of FPL), subsidies disappear, while mandatory premiums would increase to $10,585, with OOP costs capped at $6,250.[9,10]

NerdWallet, a financial-advice company, adds further perspective to medical debt in this country. In a 2014 report, it found that Americans pay three times more for medical debt than for bank and credit-card debt combined, and that almost one in five of us will be contacted by medical debt collectors each year.[11] According to the Consumer Financial Protection Bureau, an estimated 43 million people have an account in collection for medical debt.[12]

Why Medical Bankruptcy Continues Beyond the ACA

The ACA did try to ameliorate this problem by setting up insurance exchanges, enacting annual and lifetime caps on medical expenses, and expanding Medicaid. But as we saw in the last chapter, these provisions leave many holes in the system, with rising health care prices and medical debt continuing as major problems.

To better understand why medical debt and bankruptcy will continue, and perhaps even increase, under the ACA, we first need to look at the broader economic picture. The 2015 Milliman Medical Index (MMI) gives us this picture for a typical American family of four covered by an average employer-sponsored preferred provider organization (PPO) plan today:

- The cost of health care for a typical family of four covered by an average employer-sponsored PPO plan in 2015 is $24,671; this will exceed $25,000 in 2016.
- The median annual income for American households in 2015 is about $53,800.
- Costs for the typical family of four have doubled over the last decade.
- Over the last 10 years, the consumer price index has grown by about 3.3 percent a year, compared to an MMI increase of 7.3 percent a year.
- Prescription drug costs increased by 13.6 percent from 2014 to 2015.[13]
- The ACA's annual caps on OOP spending does not protect insured from out-of-network costs.
- Because of the high costs of cancer drugs and care, patients with cancer in the U.S. are more than twice as likely to declare bankruptcy as patients with other diseases.[14]

The Economic Policy Institute has developed a Family Budget Calculator as a way for families to measure annual income needed to live free of serious economic deprivation. Based on 2014 data in its updated 2015 report, Figure 12.1 puts these numbers in perspective in terms of the reality of major average costs of living for various types of families, including the seven basic components of family budgets—housing, food, transportation, child care, health care, other necessities, and taxes. The basic family budget for a family of four ranges from $49,114 in Morristown, Tenn. to $106,493 in Washington, D.C., with a median family budget of $63,741 in Des Moines, Iowa, all well above the 2014 poverty threshold of $24,008 for this family type.[15]

FIGURE 12.1

MONTHLY FAMILY BUDGETS IN DES MOINES, IOWA,* BY FAMILY TYPE, 2014

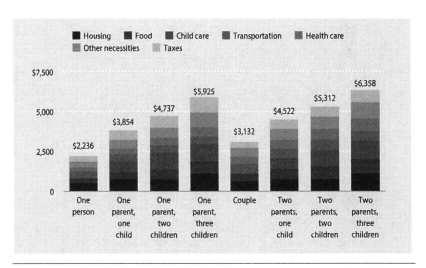

* Des Moines, Iowa is the median family budget area for a two-parent, two-child family.

Source: EPI Family Budget calculator.[15]

By these measures, it is obvious that health care has priced itself way beyond the means of ordinary Americans.

Returning to the ACA, it becomes clear why it cannot hope to address this widening disconnect between Americans' needs for health care and their ability as Americans to afford it, *even when they are insured.* These are some of the main reasons for pessimism on this count, as we have seen in earlier chapters:

- There are no significant price controls throughout our largely for-profit system.
- Our safety net through Medicaid is in tatters in many states, 20 of which opted out of Medicaid expansion; many other states have very restricted eligibility and coverage policies.
- Cost-sharing for plans purchased on the exchanges continues to increase faster than peoples' capacity to afford them.
- Most enrollees in ACA plans through the exchanges get silver or bronze plans, with actuarial values of only 70 and 60 percent, respectively.
- Pew research has shown that 55 percent of American households are savings-limited, able only to replace less than one month of their income through liquid savings.[16]

Medical bills jeopardize more than families' financial health, since families facing high medical costs are more likely to delay necessary medical care, skip filling a prescription, have worse outcomes when they do get care, and report problems paying for other necessities.[17]

Summary

Insurers are shifting ever more costs to patients and their families, while they and other industries exploit their expanded markets at taxpayer expense. We saw in the last chapter how many holes there are in the ACA's insurance plans and how extensive underinsurance is. And we will see in Chapter 15 how soaring health care costs will become even more unaffordable than today.

There is a fix—not-for-profit national health insurance (NHI), coupled with a more accountable private delivery system, as we will discuss in Part Three. NHI can eliminate the medical bankruptcy problem, rein in prices, reduce bureaucracy, and cost us far less than we are paying today. Medical bankruptcies are rare or non-existent in other countries with universal coverage policies, as T. R. Reid described in his important book, *The Healing of America: A Global Quest for Better, Cheaper and Fairer Health Care.* Meanwhile, until we develop the political will to enact such a program, we are still burdened by what Sen. Edward Kennedy called "the double disaster—the shadow of combined financial ruin and illness."[18]

References:

1. Walker, J. Actually, Obama, your health care law will not stop medical bankruptcy. *Shadow Proof*, April 30, 2013.
2. Santich, K. Despite insurance, medical bills push family to bankruptcy. *Orlando Sentinel,* July 30, 2011.
3. Himmelstein, DU, Warren, E, Thorne, D et al. Illness and injury as contributors to bankruptcy. *Health Affairs*, February 2, 2005.
4. Himmelstein, DU, Thorne, D, Warren, E et al. Medical bankruptcy in the United States, 2007: results of a national study. *Amer J Med* 122 (8): 741-746, 2009.
5. Himmelstein, DU, Woolhandler, S. Medical bankruptcy in Massachusetts: has health reform made a difference? *Amer J Med* 124 (3): 224-228, 2011.
6. Farley, PJ. Who are the underinsured? *Milbank Q* 63: 476-503, 1985.
7. Farley, PJ, Short, P, Banthin, JS. New estimates of the underinsured younger than 65 years. *JAMA* 274: 1302-1306, 1995.
8. Collins, SR, Doty, MM, Robertson, R et al. Help on the horizon: findings from the Commonwealth Fund Biennial Health Insurance Survey of 2010. *The Commonwealth Fund.* Washington, D.C., March 2011.
9. The Henry J. Kaiser Family Foundation. Health reform subsidy calculator. Available at: http://healthreform.kff.org/subsidycalculator.aspx
10. Woolhandler, S, Himmelstein, DU. Life or debt: underinsurance in America. *J Gen Intern Med,* published on line, April 25, 2013.
11. Khazan, O. Why Americans are drowning in medical debt. *The Atlantic,* October 8, 2014.
12. Hillebrand, G. Consumer Advisory: 7 ways to keep medical debt in check. *Consumer Financial Protection Bureau,* December 11, 2014.
13. Milliman. 2015 Milliman Medical Index. May 2015.
14. Ramsey, S, Blough, D, Kirchhoff, A et al. Washington State cancer patients found to be at greater risk of bankruptcy than people without a cancer diagnosis. Health Affairs (Millwood) 32 (6): 1143-1152, 2013.
15. Gould, E, Cooke, T, Kimball, W. What families need to get by: EPI's 2015 Family Budget Calculator. Economic Policy Institute, August 26, 2015.

16. Pew Charitable Trusts. The precarious state of family balance sheets. January 29, 2015.
17. Himmelstein, DU, Woolhandler, S. Medical debt: a curable affliction health reform won't fix. *Communities & Banking*, Federal Reserve Bank of Boston, Summer 2013.
18. Ibid # 17.

PART TWO

System Trends Under the Affordable Care Act

The ACA set the stage for a financial boon for the health care industry in numerous ways. It enables millions of new customers to purchase individual policies. It permits Medicaid programs in many states to retain more managed care companies to administer benefits. It helps hospitals and many physicians to realize increased revenues by giving more of their patients access to the financial resources needed to pay for care. And, over time, countless other businesses will emerge and thrive under the ACA's government-created structure as the ingenuity of the private sector finds ways to thrive off its new public base.[1]

—Robert Field, professor of law and of health policy and
management at Drexel University and author of *Mother
of Invention: How the Government Created
"Free-Market" Health Care*

Reference:

1. Field, RI. *Mother of Invention: How the Government Created "Free-Market" Health Care*. New York. *Oxford University Press*, 2014, pp. 220-221.

The Myth: Consolidation brings more efficiency, more competition and lowers costs.

CHAPTER 13

MORE CONSOLIDATION, *LESS* COMPETITION

The ACA has fueled a merger frenzy among corporate giants in the medical-industrial complex, accelerated since the U.S. Supreme Court's 2015 ruling in favor of subsidies in the federal exchanges. A number of billion-dollar deals have taken place as health insurers, hospitals and drug companies position themselves to profit from increased government spending on the ACA's exchanges, state Medicaid programs and Medicare Advantage for the baby boomers. Gerald Kominski, director of the UCLA Center for Health Policy Research, brings us this insight:

> *The Affordable Care Act is driving this merger mania. There are billions of dollars pouring into the system, and it's money to buy insurance.*[1]

Just halfway through calendar year 2015, about $2.15 trillion of merger-and-acquisition (M & A) deals were announced globally, according to Dealogic. The CEOs of many companies seem to fear being left behind by rivals and becoming takeover prey themselves. Previously, 2007 had been the record year for M & A deals, at $4.3 trillion, and 2015 is on track to surpass that. Later in 2015, Allergen, with a current market value of $113 billion with an offshore headquarters in Dublin, was in talks to merge with Pfizer, while Walgreens Boots Alliance announced its purchase of Rite Aid, creating a chain of more than 12,000 U. S. pharmacies, and CVS acquired Omnicare to expand its reach into nursing homes.[2] The health care sector has led the way in these mergers compared to the other four top sectors: oil and gas, technology, telecom, and real estate/property.[3]

The mantra of market ideology, of course, holds that bigger is better, that consolidation will bring more efficiency, and that more competition should lower costs for consumers. Though recent years cast doubt on these claims, let's try to sort through what is happening across the health care industries and what their impacts on all of us are likely to be.

Accelerating Mergers in Health Care Industries

Let's look at two of the biggest industries in the medical-industrial complex to see what's actually happening.

1. The Insurance Industry

Consolidation is being driven by insurers' response to a shifting health insurance market as an ever-larger share of their market is tied to growing government programs and the exchanges under the ACA. Since 2005, percentage changes in annual enrollments have increased 52 percent for Medicaid, 31 percent for Medicare, and 25 percent for individual coverage, while employer-sponsored insurance dropped by 3.5 percent.[4]

Though it is easy for us to ascribe all of these changes to the ACA, as Republicans are wont to do, there is a larger context to this trend. Wendell Potter, executive at Cigna for many years before becoming a whistleblower against the industry and writing his important book, *Deadly Spin: An Insurance Company Insider Speaks Out on How Corporate PR is Killing Health Care and Deceiving Americans,* reminds us that major consolidation of health insurers took place in the mid-to late 1990s in order to gain more leverage in negotiating with hospitals and physician groups. (Ironically, that consolidation later drove self-defense consolidation on the provider side, thus increasing the stakes). Potter also notes the role of demographic changes in altering the insurance marketplace, especially the aging of baby boomers and a growing Medicare market. The declining role of ESI has had a negative impact on the two leading insurers in that area—Cigna and Aetna—further roiling the insurance markets.[5]

These two big deals were agreed to in mid-2015, and are now in process, subject to approval by shareholders and regulators:

- Aetna acquires Humana for $37 billion in cash and stock in a deal that will close in the second half of 2016. The combined company is expected to generate more than one-half of its revenues from Medicare and Medicaid markets.[6]
- Anthem buys its big rival, Cigna, for $54.2 billion, the largest such merger in U.S. history, which will, if finalized, reduce the number of major insurers from five to three. The merged company is projected to cover 53 million people, mostly in the employer-based and individual markets.[7]

It is possible that regulators may try to block some of the growing numbers of mergers. Antitrust officials at the Justice Department and the Federal Trade Commission (FTC) are increasingly concerned that these mergers can hurt consumers. And the Anthem-Cigna deal raises complexities with the Blue Cross and Blue Shield brand names, which Anthem has used as a major way of becoming the nation's second-largest health insurer.[8] At this writing, it appears that just three health insurance giants will soon dominate the market more than ever before, as shown by Table 13.1.[9] Already, a recent report from the Commonwealth Fund has found that 97 percent of markets for private Medicare plans in U.S. counties are "highly concentrated," with little competition.[10]

Insurers tell us to trust them—that mergers will enable them to operate more efficiently and negotiate more effectively with other large players, such as hospital systems and drug companies.

TABLE 13.1

THREE HEALTH INSURANCE GIANTS

INSURER	COMBINED MEMBERSHIP	PROJECTED 2015 REVENUE	STRENGTHS
Anthem/Cigna	53.2 million	$117 billion	Biggest overall membership
UnitedHealth Group	45.8 million	$154 billion	Largest annual revenue, fueled by growing Optum health-services arm
Aetna/Humana	33.5 million	$115 billion	Biggest player in Medicare Advantage

Source: Mattioli, D, Hoffman, L, Mathews, AW. Anthem nears $48 billion Cigna deal. *Wall Street Journal*, July 23, 2015:A1.

Meanwhile, not surprisingly, the intense interest by Wall Street in these mergers is illustrated by the New York-based hedge fund, Glenview Capital Management LLC, which over the last four years has invested heavily in Humana, Anthem, Aetna, and Cigna. With these deals, this fund achieved increases in stock prices ranging from 23 percent for Anthem to 50 percent for Cigna, thereby making realized and paper gains of more than $3.2 billion.[11] So much for the ACA being a federal takeover, squashing the private sector!

2. The Hospital Industry

Growth and consolidation of hospital systems has been going on for a long time. As of 2014, the three largest for-profit hospital chains in the U.S. were: Community Health Systems, based in Franklin, Tennessee with 191 hospitals; Nashville, TN based Hospital Corporation of America with 160 hospitals; and Dallas, Texas based Tenet Healthcare Corp. with 72 hospitals.[12]

It is not just that these expanding hospital systems consolidate with larger market shares, but also that they buy up physician group practices and thereby control large parts of medical practice in their areas. With less competition, prices for outpatient care predictably go up, as documented by a recent study.[13] The FTC has been very concerned about this trend. Basing its challenges on the century-old Clayton Antitrust Act of 1914, it is winning big cases. As director of the FTC's bureau of economics, Martin S. Gaynor, has this to say:

> *Hospitals that face less competition charge substantially higher prices . . . as much as 40 to 50 percent higher.*[14]

As insurers as payers and hospitals/medical groups as providers expand and consolidate, they are bulking up to seek more leverage in contract negotiations. Robert Kocher, a former White House health advisor now at the venture-capital firm, Venrock, observes:

> *The ACA is a trigger. Payers have been finding that they're getting pushed by providers saying 'Take my rates or you'll have no network.'*[15]

Impacts of Consolidation on Patients and Families

Despite the theories and ideology of private markets being more efficient and competitive, consolidation does not work that way. The more consolidation, the more oligopoly reigns and the easier it is for corporate giants to raise prices to what the traffic will bear. Let's see how this plays out in two health industries.

Private insurers

As insurers gain commanding market shares in their part of the insurance market, and in their geographic areas, they follow their business plans and corporate self-interest at the expense of their enrollees. The three consolidated insurers shown in Table 13.1 are on a path to control almost one-half of the commercial health insurance market in the U.S. In that capacity, they can charge premiums with less regard for competitors, and may have a stronger hand in negotiating lower prices from hospitals and physician groups. In addition, they reduce patients' choices of hospitals and providers as they narrow their networks, as Martin Gaynor points out:

> *While it is possible that a giant insurer battling a giant hospital system could lead to lower prices—because the insurer is able to extract lower prices from the large health system—the benefits may not necessarily flow to consumers. . . [In a market with two behemoths] consumers are left on the outside looking in.*[16]

Academy Health is a leading national organization involved in health services and health policy research. It issued a recent report based on a study by an expert panel that examined the impacts of narrow networks and tiered networks on consumers. The report raised serious concerns about narrow networks being established by insurers, including these:

> *Unless risk adjustment accounts for differences in patient mix and health status is employed and working well, the constructions of narrow networks could be used to discriminate against patients with complex conditions and greater needs. . . Questions about the effectiveness of risk adjustment remain unanswered. . . . There is a need for greater oversight of and better standards to measure network adequacy.*[157]

Commenting on this study, Dr. Don McCanne, senior health policy fellow for Physicians for a National Health Program, has this to say:

As this report indicates, insurers select their network providers base on the lowest prices that they can negotiate—not on quality. . . The only advantage that the insurers can tout is that patients allegedly are paying less in premiums and cost sharing because of the lower rates that insurers were able to negotiate on their behalf. But the private insurers are an intrusion that are responsible for not only their own expensive administrative excesses but also for the profound and costly administrative burden that they place on the health care delivery system. . . . Since these administrative costs are far greater than the negotiated discounts they receive from providers, the insurers are actually increasing costs for patients.[18]

Dr. David Himmelstein, professor of public health at the City University of New York and visiting professor of medicine at Harvard Medical School, adds this important insight:

[This latest wave of mergers] will turn insurance giants into 'essential monopolies' that make a significant profit from public tax dollars. Much of their revenue comes from the government that pays hundreds of billions annually in premiums for private Medicare Advantage plans, Medicaid managed care plans, and much of the premiums for the private plans bought on [ACA] insurance exchanges. Much of this money is wasted; Anthem and Cigna have overhead that's nearly tenfold higher than traditional Medicare.[19]

Many studies have documented that insurance mergers lead to higher premiums, especially as larger insurers crowd out smaller ones. As just one example, a 2009 analysis of a 1999 merger between Aetna and Prudential found that real premiums rose by about 7 percent in a typical market due to increased concentration, and that there was a tendency to cut employees and substitute nurses for physicians.[20]

Hospitals

Can we expect anything better as hospitals further consolidate? The answer is clearly no, as shown by a 2015 report of a study of the 50 highest-charging for-profit hospitals in the country. These hospitals have markups about *ten times higher* than Medicare-allowable costs! They are concentrated in Florida, and one-half are owned by a single chain. Among all U.S. hospitals, the average markup is 3.4 times higher than Medicare-allowable costs.[21] Gerald Anderson, professor of health policy at Johns Hopkins Bloomberg School of Public Health and one of the authors of this study, tells us that:

> *For the most part, there is no regulation of hospital rates and there are no market forces that force hospitals to lower their rates. They charge these prices simply because they can.*[22]

As hospital systems expand and further consolidate, they typically buy up physician groups in their areas. This leads to the probability that employed physicians will admit patients to their employers' hospitals, which often are higher-cost, lower-quality hospitals. A recent study by researchers at Stanford University found that physicians employed by hospitals admitted an average of 83 percent of their hospitalized patients to their proprietor hospital.[23]

Summary

As we can see, consolidation is increasing across health insurance companies and hospital systems, spurred on even more by the ACA, with no significant regulation in sight. Private interests are exploiting new, expanded markets, enabled by government policies and subsidies that we as patients and taxpayers pay for. The corporate giants in the medical-industrial complex are winners, as are Wall Street and investors, but all at the expense of patients and their families. In the next chapter, we will look at another growing threat to the public interest in health care.

References:

1. Terhune, C. Obamacare cash fuels healthcare merger mania. *Los Angeles Times*, July 2, 2015.
2. Abelson, R. Health care companies in merger frenzy. *New York Times*, October 29, 2015.
3. Mattioli, D, Camilluca, D. Fear of losing out drives deal boom. *Wall Street Journal*, June 27, 2015: A1.
4. Cimilluca, D, Mattioli, Mathews, AW. Medical insurers on prowl for deals. *Wall Street Journal*, June 16, 2015: A1.
5. Potter, W. GOP myth: Obamacare is driving insurance mergers. *The Progressive Populist*, August 15, 2015.
6. Bray, C, Abelson, R. Aetna agrees to acquire Humana for $37 billion in cash and stock. *New York Times,* July 3, 2015.
7. Lazare, S. Healthcare 'oligopoly wave' continues as Anthem gobbles Cigna. *Common Dreams*, July 24, 2015.
8. Wall, JK. Anthem-Cigna mega deal might snag on Blue Cross. *Indianapolis Business Journal*, August 8, 2015.
9. Mattioli, Hofman, L, Mathews, AW. Anthem nears $48 billion Cigna deal. *Wall Street Journal*, July 23, 2015: A1.
10. Abelson, R. With mergers, concerns grow about private Medicare. *New York Times*, August 25, 2015.
11. Benoit, D. Fund boss's gamble on health law paid off big. *Wall Street Journal*, July 24, 2015: A 1.
12. Top 10 U.S. for-profit hospital operators based on number of hospitals as of 2014. *The Statistics Portal* htpp://www.statista.com/statistics/245010/top-us-for-profit-hospi…
13. Neprash, HT, Chernew, ME, Hicks, SL et al. Association of financial integration with commercial health care prices. *JAMA Internal Medicine*, October 19, 2015.
14. Pear, R. F.T.C. wary of mergers by hospitals. *New York Times*, September 17, 2014.
15. Mathews, AW. Health law speeds merger frenzy. *Wall Street Journal*, September 22, 2015: B1.

16. Abelson, R. Bigger may be better for health insurers, but doubts remain for consumers. *New York Times*, August 2, 2015.
17. Summer, L. Health plan features: implications of narrow networks and the trade-off between price and choice. *Academy Health Research Insights*, April 3, 2015.
18. McCanne, D. Ibid # 16, commentary. April 3, 2015.
19. Himmelstein, DU. As quoted by Ibid # 4.
20. Dafny, L, Duggan, M, Ramanarayanan, S. Paying a premium on your premium? Consolidation in the U.S. health insurance industry. NBER Working Paper No. 15434. *National Bureau of Economic Research.* Washington, D.C., October 2009.
21. Bai, G, Anderson, GF. Extreme markup: the fifty U.S. hospitals with the highest charge-to-cost ratios. *Health Affairs* 34 (6): 922-928, June 2015.
22. Anderson, G. As quoted by Gold, J. Study: Highest-charging U.S. hospitals are for-profits, concentrated in Florida. *Kaiser Health News*, June 8, 2015.
23. Hancock, J. When the hospital is boss, that's where doctors' patients go. *Kaiser Health News,* September 9, 2015.

Myth: Privatized health care is more efficient, offers more choice and better value.

CHAPTER 14

INCREASING PRIVATIZATION

No other nation expects a private sector, little constrained by public rules on the size and terms of employer contributions, to carry so heavy a burden of coverage, and none asks private insurers to hold the line with providers (including specialists, uncommonly abundant in the United States) on prices outside a framework of public policies that guide the bargaining game. The first of these two grand exceptions largely accounts for the nation's high rates of un- and underinsurance; the latter mainly explains why American health spending is so high by cross-national standards.[1]

—Lawrence Brown, professor of health policy
and management at Columbia University

There has been a long-held belief that private markets, left to their own devices with minimal regulation, can and will solve affordability and distribution challenges. This goes back to the concept of the "invisible hand," a term coined by Adam Smith in 1759, before the advent of economics as a discipline, whereby free markets would work in everyone's best interests. This idea still has wide cultural appeal in this country, and is endorsed without critique by many conservatives, economists, and policymakers. But, as we have already seen in this book, our market-based system has been unable to redress serious problems of access, costs, affordability, and quality of health care for our population.

As Joseph Stiglitz, professor of economics at Columbia University and Nobel laureate in economics, has observed:

> *Adam Smith, the father of modern economics, is often cited as arguing for the 'invisible hand' and free markets. But unlike his followers, Adam Smith was aware of some of the limitations of free markets, and research since then has further clarified why free markets, by themselves, often do not lead to what is best . . . [The] reason that the invisible hand often seems invisible is that it is often not there.*[2]

The ACA was crafted to serve the interests of private corporate stakeholders, enabled by what turns out to be a naïve belief among the ACA's architects that private markets can be re-directed for the public good. Some who were closely involved in the politics of U.S. health care over recent years saw this coming. Tom Scully, former administrator of CMS during the George W. Bush administration, had this to say as the keynote speaker at a meeting of the Potomac Research Group, a Beltway firm that advises large investors on government policy:

> *Obamacare is not a government takeover of medicine. It is the privatization of health care. . . . It's going to make some people very rich.*[3]

This chapter has two goals: (1) to trace the growing role of privatization of Medicare over the last 50 years in this country, and (2) to summarize the adverse impacts of privatized Medicare and Medicaid programs on patients and their families as well as taxpayers.

Historical Perspective: A Long Push to Privatize U.S. Health Care

The last 50 years have seen a remarkable paradigm shift in how we as a society have viewed and dealt with the health care needs of the vulnerable among us. By the early 1960s, most seniors were unable to afford health insurance. Insurers often refused coverage to people based on pre-existing conditions, and if they offered coverage, would charge older enrollees five or ten times more than younger people for the same policies.

In response, Medicare was passed in 1965 as the first program of publicly financed social insurance, covering 10 percent of our population, with overwhelming bipartisan support in Congress—by votes of 302-116 in the House and 70-24 in the Senate. Medicaid was passed the same year as a means to provide a safety net to enable lower-income Americans to have access to necessary health care. Both programs have since become part of the fabric of American life.

Since the 1960s, however, there have been incremental pressures by conservative interests (in both political parties) to privatize these social programs. Those efforts started earlier for Medicare than for Medicaid.

Privatization of Medicare

During the Nixon administration in 1972, Social Security amendments were enacted authorizing Medicare to contract with private HMOs on a capitation basis, with requirements that participating plans would be subject to retrospective cost adjustments and constraints upon their profits; by 1979, only one plan had signed up.[4]

Amid growing concerns among policymakers about the rising costs of Medicare, Congress passed the Tax Equity and Fiscal Responsibility Act of 1982 (TEFRA), which authorized Medicare to contract with HMOs and pay them 95 percent of traditional Medicare's adjusted average per capita cost in each county of the U.S. The original idea was that Medicare HMOs would save money, but that 95 percent figure later morphed to much more—up to 115 percent or even more than the costs of traditional Medicare in overpayments.

The early and mid-1990s were prosperous years for Medicare HMOs (then called Medicare + Choice), peaking in 1998 with enrollment of about 17 percent of Medicare beneficiaries. When Republicans gained control of both houses of Congress in 1994, there was a vigorous new push to privatize Medicare. It was argued that the long-term financial viability was at risk, especially with future enrollments of the baby boomer generation, and that private markets are more efficient. With the Balanced Budget Act of 1995, the new House Majority introduced a plan to completely privatize Medicare, shifting it from a defined benefits to defined contribution program. Then Speaker of the House Newt Gingrich predicted that this kind of "reform" would "solve the Medicare problem" by causing it "to wither on the vine."[5] While it did not pass in Congress, the 1997 Balanced Budget Act (BBA 97) was later passed, cutting annual payment increases for most Medicare HMOs to 2 percent a year, prompting their large-scale exodus from the market as they lost their generous (and unearned) overpayments.[6]

Conservative policymakers, backed by such conservative think tanks as the Heritage Foundation, kept up the pressure to replace Medicare as "an entitlement program" with a system wherein all beneficiaries would pay their own way in a "more efficient" private system. They also continued to lobby for higher overpayments and lesser regulation of Medicare HMOs.

The next big move to more privatization came with the Medicare Prescription Drug, Improvement and Modernization Act of 2003 (MMA), full of provisions that increase cost sharing, limit some benefits, and subsidize the private sector. It was a bonanza for the insurance and pharmaceutical industries, even including a federal bonus subsidy of $1.3 billion, to be paid during 2004 and 2005 and estimated to be about 120 percent of what Medicare pays for traditional coverage.[7]

Fast forward to recent times and we see the same arguments and political pressure to further privatize Medicare, in a continuing effort to extract more profits from a federal program. H.R. 2, the Medicare Access and CHIP Reauthorization Act of 2015 (MA-CRA), was passed by Congress after heated debate and horse-trading between the two parties. Very complex and still poorly understood, it did eliminate the Sustainable Growth Rate formula (SGR) that tied physician payments to economic growth and led to recurrent budget crises since its enactment in 1997. It enacts different ways to pay physicians with new incentives intended to contain costs and improve quality of care.[8] But these new incentives are very unlikely to contain future costs, and will lead to more gaming of the new system by providers. H.R. 2 also introduces means-testing for higher-income beneficiaries, thus further breaking up Medicare's original social contract.

During this 2016 election cycle, here is what former Florida Governor Jeb Bush, as a presidential candidate on the campaign trail, said in this disjointed comment about Medicare:

> *We need to make sure we fulfill the commitment to people that have already received the benefits, that are receiving the benefits. But we need to figure out a way to phase out this program for others and move to a new system that allows them to have something, because they're not going to have anything.*[9]

In July 2015, on the 50th anniversary of Medicare and Medicaid, the two programs combined covered more than one-third of Americans. Many of these were in privatized programs—more than 30 percent of Medicare's 55 million beneficiaries and well over one-half of Medicaid's 66 million enrollees. These enrollments, especially for Medicaid, have soared since the ACA expanded Medicaid.[10] By 2014, there were 267 mostly for-profit managed Medicaid programs (MMC) across the country.[11] In a recent merger, Centene acquired Health Net, and plans to become one of the largest Medicaid insurers in the country.[12]

What's So Wrong with Privatized Health Care?

Privatized Medicare

Compared to traditional Medicare, privatized Medicare is:
1. more expensive,
2. less efficient,
3. less reliable,
4. more restrictive choice of physician and hospital, and
5. has higher administrative costs.

Table 14.1 shows the marked differences between traditional Medicare and private Medicare plans.[13]

TABLE 14.1

COMPARATIVE FEATURES OF PRIVATIZED AND PUBLIC MEDICARE

PRIVATIZED MEDICARE	ORIGINAL MEDICARE
Experience-rated eligibility	Universal coverage
Managed competition	Social insurance as earned right
Defined contribution	Defined benefits
Segmented risk pool	Broad risk pool
Market pricing to risk	Administered prices
More volatile access & benefits	More reliable access & benefits
Increased cost sharing	Less cost sharing
Less accountability	Potential for more accountability
Less choice of provider & hospital	Full choice of provider & hospital
Less well distributed	Well distributed
Less efficiency, higher overhead	More efficiency, lower overhead

Source: Geyman, JP. *Shredding the Social Contract The Privatization of Medicare.* Monroe, ME. *Common Courage Press*, 2006, p.206

According to this study by the Commonwealth Fund in 2001, traditional Medicare is rated more highly than private insurance by five criteria as shown in Figure 14.1.[14]

FIGURE 14.1

MEDICARE COVERAGE IS BETTER THAN PRIVATE

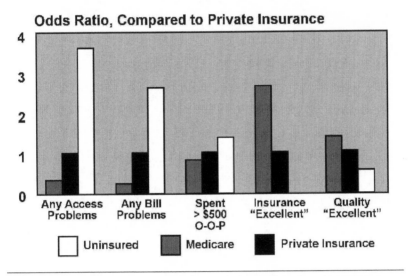

Reprinted with permission from Physicians for a National Health Program (PNHP), Source: Davis K. Medicare versus private insurance: rhetoric and reality. *Health Affairs Web Exclusive*, Oct. 9, 2002, W311-23

Fee-for-service Medicare has also been shown to contain health care costs better than privatized Medicare over the 30-year period 1970 to 2000 (Figure 14.2)[15] Traditional Medicare's comparative effectiveness in cost containment is attributed to its low overhead and its ability to set prices for the services it covers.[16]

Privatized Medicaid

Although privatized Medicaid has a shorter history than privatized Medicare, it shares many of the same kinds of problems, including high administrative costs, built-in profits, restricted choice, and more volatility. These are some examples of the downsides of privatized Medicaid programs:

FIGURE 14.2

CUMULATIVE GROWTH IN PER ENROLLEE PAYMENTS FOR PERSONAL HEALTH CARE MEDICARE AND PRIVATE INSURERS, 1970-2000

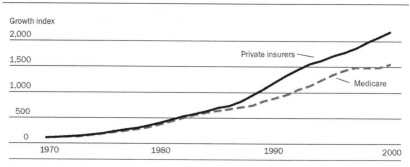

Sources: Urban Institute analysis of National Health Accounts data from the Centers for Medicare and Medicaid Services; Boccuti, C, Moon, M. Comparing Medicare and private insurers: growth rates in spending over three decades. *Health Affairs (Millwood)* 22 (2): 230, 2003. Reprinted with permission.

- Tennessee Medicaid plans, operated by BlueCross BlueShield of Tennessee, UnitedHealthcare, and Anthem, illustrate the inadequacies of MMC plans, with inadequate physician networks, long waits for care, and denials of many treatments, even as the insurers pocket new profits.[17]
- Typical Medicaid reimbursement is only 61 percent of what Medicare pays for the same service; as a result, only one-third of health care providers are accepting Medicaid patients.[18]
- Some states have received federal waivers to impose premiums and/or copays to Medicaid patients; this cost-sharing has been shown to result in disenrollment and decreased access to care.[19]
- Subcontracting of Medicaid coverage has almost doubled Medicaid's administrative overhead, increasing from 5.1 percent of total Medicaid expenditures in 1980 to 9.2 percent today.[20]

Summary

Cost containment in a largely for-profit market-based system is a mirage, a cruel delusion, despite the continuing rhetoric from the right and a compliant middle of the political debate over health care. The difference is simple—markets follow a business model, which is in conflict with the public interest. The last 40 years should have taught us this lesson. Will we ever learn and start to recognize what all other advanced countries discovered long ago—that a larger role of government is required to meet the needs of populations for affordable access to necessary health care?

The ACA, crafted as it was to serve the interests of corporate stakeholders in the private sector, cut a Faustian bargain with them. The Obama administration *needs* the full participation of private insurers in order to claim expanded insurance access, but is dependent on keeping them happy. Thus, whenever cutting overpayments to Medicare Advantage comes up, there is a firestorm of protest in Congress to "not do anything to hurt Grandma's Medicare", and the overpayments continue. Recall the exodus of Medicare + Choice HMOs in the late 1990s in reaction to cuts at that time.

Dr. Arnold Relman, the late internist and former editor of *The New England Journal of Medicine,* was right on target with this observation ten years ago:

> *U.S. health policies have failed to meet national needs during the past four decades because they have been heavily influenced by the delusion that medical care is essentially a business. . . . The current rate of inflation in health care costs is unsustainable, and it is likely that any market-based solutions will fail to address the problem. . . . A real solution to our crisis will not be found until the public, the medical profession, and the government reject the prevailing delusion that health care is best left to market forces.*[21]

References:

1. Brown, LD. In Stevens, RA, Rosenberg, CE, Burns, LR (eds) *History and Health Policy in the United States: Putting the Past Back In*. New Brunswick, NJ. *Rutgers University Press*, 2006: 46.

2. Stiglitz, J. As cited by Matthews, C. The 'invisible hand' has an iron grip on America. *Fortune*, August 13, 2014.

3. Scully, T. As cited by Davidson, A. The President wants you to get rich on Obamacare. *The New York Times Magazine*, October 30, 2013.

4. Oberlander, JB. Managed care and Medicare reform. *J Health Polit. Policy Law* 595: 598, 1997.

5. Gingrich, N. As cited by Smith, DG. *Entitlement Politics: Medicare and Medicaid 1995-2001*. New York. Aldine de Gruyter, 2002: 71, citing *Congressional Quarterly Almanac*, 1995, pp. 7-13.

6. Pretzer, M. Medicare: the managed care program isn't working the way Congress intended. *Med Econ*, June 19, 2003, p. 31.

7. Headstart for HMOs: *Medicare Watch* 6 (25): 2, 2003.

8. Aaron, HJ. Three cheers for logrolling: the demise of the SGR. *Health360, Brookings*, April 22, 2015.

9. Bush, J. As quoted by Potter, W. Privatizing Medicare would create more problems than it solves. *Center for Public Integrity*, August 3, 2015.

10. Pear, R. As Medicare and Medicaid turn 50, use of private health plans surges. *New York Times*, July 30, 2015: A12.

11. Tavernise, S, Gebeloff, R. Millions of poor are left uncovered by health law. *New York Times*, October 2, 1013.

12. Terhune, C. Obamacare cash fuels healthcare merger mania. *Los Angeles Times*, July 2, 2015.

13. Geyman, JP. *Shredding the Social Contract: The Privatization of Medicare*. Monroe, ME. *Common Courage Press*, 2006, p. 206.

14. Davis, K. Medicare versus private insurance: rhetoric and reality. *Health Affairs Web Exclusive*, October 9, 2002, W311-323.

15. Boccuti, C, Moon, M. Comparing Medicare and private insurers: growth rates in spending over three decades. *Health Affairs (Millwood)* 22 (2): 230, 2003.

16. Bodenheimer, T. *The Dismal Failure of Medicare Privatization,* p. 18. *Senior Action Network,* San Francisco, June 2003.
17. Himmelstein, DU, Woolhandler, S. The post-launch problem: the Affordable Care Act's persistently high administrative costs. *Health Affairs Blog,* May 27, 2015.
18. Coleman, K. Medicaid acceptance by healthcare providers drops to 1-out-of-3. *HealthPocket,* February 26, 2015.
19. Levy, N. Four largest states have sharp disparities in access to health care. *Los Angeles Times*, April 10, 2015.
20. Ibid # 17.
21. Relman, AS. The health of nations. *The New Republic.* March 7, 2005.

Myth: Market competition lowers costs.

CHAPTER 15

SOARING COSTS AND PATIENTS PAY MORE

I find little evidence anywhere that market forces, bluntly used, that is, consumer choice among an array of products with competitors fighting it out, leads to the health care system you want and need. In the U.S. competition has become toxic: it is a major reason for our duplicative, supply-driven, fragmented health care system. . . . Unfettered growth and pursuit of institutional self-interest has been the engine of low value for the U.S. health care system. It has made it unaffordable, and hasn't helped patients at all.[1]

—Dr. Donald Berwick, former president and
CEO of the Institute for Health Care Improvement and
former Administrator of the Centers for Medicare
and Medicaid Services (CMS)

Yes, "competition" in U.S. health care has become toxic, at least for patients, as we saw also in Chapter 13 on consolidating corporate players. Despite the drum beat from market interests that competition is alive, well, and reducing costs, it is time to recognize this as a myth and look for other ways to control costs of health care. As Phil Caper, M.D., Maine internist with long experience in health policy dating back to the 1970s, observes:

Our profit-driven health care system is bankrupting individuals, putting enormous stress on businesses and state and federal governments and destroying the therapeutic doctor-patient bond of trust.[2]

This chapter has three goals: (1) to summarize the extent and reasons for continuing inflation of health care costs; (2) to show the impacts of these costs as so many people with stagnant incomes struggle to afford care; and (3) to compare health care costs in this country versus other advanced countries and ask if any effective cost containment approaches are yet in sight.

Relentless Inflation of Health Care Costs

As just one among many examples of research finding the lack of real competition in health care, the non-profit Center for Studying Health System Change (HSC) carried out an eight-year Community Tracking Study (CTS) tracking change in 12 randomly selected, nationally representative metropolitan communities (Boston, Cleveland, Greenville, SC, Indianapolis, Lansing, Little Rock, Miami, northern New Jersey, Orange County, CA, Phoenix, Seattle, and Syracuse, NY). Its 2004 report found that:

1. Providers had enough market power in most sites to set their own prices, dictate the terms of their arrangements with health plans, and sidestep pressures to provide technically efficient care.
2. Most physician markets were so fragmented that the potential efficiencies of integrated delivery systems were not achievable.
3. Employers lacked the clout to push their local systems toward efficiency and quality.
4. There was insufficient health plan competition to engender more efficient local health care systems.

The final overall conclusion of the CTS was: "Based on repeated site visits to the same twelve communities, the path to a more efficient health care system is blocked by a lack of effective competition among providers."[3]

The problem of uncontrolled prices, usually not transparent, permeates our entire health care system. As hospitals buy up medical groups, clinical laboratories, imaging centers, and other outpatient facilities, their prices immediately go up. Overbilling by hospitals is common, and up-coding of physician services is epidemic.[4]

Here are other examples across the medical-industrial complex that illustrate how pervasive and inevitable continuing uncontrolled inflation of health care costs has become:

- *Insurers*—The ACA has a reinsurance program designed to protect insurers from insurance costs for sicker patients. Blue Cross organizations received large payments in 2015 even as they hiked their rates; as one example, Blue Cross Blue Shield, the largest insurer in North Carolina, received almost $295 million in federal payouts as it was seeking a 25.7 average rate increase for its individual policies.[5]
- *Hospitals*— Wide variation of charges is the norm; one example—charges for a routine appendectomy in California have ranged from $1,500 to $182,955.[6]
- *Providers' separate fees*—as insurers try to limit their costs, providers increasingly are imposing separate fees on patients, such as separate "refraction fees" for an eye exam or a "noncritical activation fee" for a trauma team in an emergency room.[7]
- *Stand-alone emergency rooms*—These are sprouting up all over the country as revenue centers, some owned by hospitals, others by physicians; they can charge double or triple what an urgent care center can[8]; free-standing ER operator Adeptus, which operates more than 60 such ERs in affluent areas of Arizona, Colorado, and Texas, (and thus can avoid Medicare and Medicaid patients in many states!), recently announced an 18 percent first-quarter jump in its stock price.[9]

- *Nursing homes*—The Inspector General's Office (OIG) of HHS has found that for-profit nursing homes, which received 78 percent of nursing home revenues in 2010, overbills Medicare by $1.5 billion a year for treatments that patients don't need or ever receive; for-profits were almost twice as likely as non-profits to bill Medicare at the highest rate for patients of similar ages and diagnoses.[10]

- *Growth of for-profits in other facilities and services*—96 percent of outpatient surgical centers are now for-profit; for-profit hospices grew ten times faster than not-for-profits from 2004 through 2009, with almost one-half now for-profit; for-profits now account for 84 percent of home health care agencies and 85 percent of dialysis clinics.[11]

- *Prescription drugs*—Prices for the 30 top-selling drugs rose almost four times as fast as prescription volume, on average from 2010 through 2014[12]; the overall cost of prescription drugs in the U.S.went up by 12 percent in the last year, the biggest annual increase in ten years; the costs of cancer drugs are among the fastest-growing, at a compound annual rate of 11.6 percent through 2020[13]; the prices of generic drugs are also soaring, partly as a result of industry consolidation and production slowdowns.[14]

- *Medical devices*— Prices of medical devices are generally not transparent, and can range widely in the same area, such as from a low of $17,000 to a high of $55,000 in Wisconsin for a total knee replacement[15]; confidentiality clauses in many medical device purchasing agreements prohibit hospitals from sharing prices with third parties, including physicians, patients, and insurers.[16]

- *Unnecessary and inappropriate care*—This is a big problem, with up to one-third of all health care services provided each year being either unnecessary or inappropriate, and some actually harmful[17]; more than 30 million full-body CT scans are performed each year for screening purposes, despite the lack of evidence for benefit or approval by the FDA or the American College of Radiology.[18]

More Cost Shifting to Patients and Less Affordability

Patients and their families are left in a very disadvantaged position as they try to cope with ongoing inflation of health care costs. In so many cases, there is no transparency of prices. Given the urgency of decisions surrounding many situations, it is not really possible for most people to "shop for the best price and value", as conservatives keep suggesting. If one is insured, that coverage is often inadequate, with changing benefits and networks, as we have seen in earlier chapters. And if one is lucky enough to have employer-sponsored insurance, employers keep shifting more costs to their employees as they try to cope with rising health care costs and look ahead to the 40 percent Cadillac tax in 2018.

When we consider how much patients and families can afford to pay for health care, we first need to recall Figure 12.1 (page 103), which shows us the major costs of living for families of four. It is obvious that there is already little room in their budgets to deal with increasing costs of insurance and health care, as we saw in some detail in Chapters 10 and 11. Many families are already dealing with financial hardship levels, as defined by the Commonwealth Fund. When we wonder how much subsidies under the ACA may be helping, we find that more than 2 million exchange enrollees are not getting subsidies because they selected a non-qualifying plan, such as a bronze plan with the lowest premiums and the lowest (60 percent) actuarial value.[19]

"Consumer driven health care" is the slogan for cost shifting to patients under the premise that "empowered" patients can make more prudent cost-conscious decisions about their own health care from the point of service on. Higher cost sharing, with increasing deductibles, copays, coinsurance, and out-of-pocket (OOP) costs is the story of our times, all to the advantage of insurers, hospital systems, the drug industry, and other parts of the medical-industrial complex. Here is just one under-the-radar example of why we can expect no improvement on the horizon without a major change in how we finance health care:

- Health care industries collectively spent $489 million on lobbying in 2014; about one-half of that was spent by the pharmaceutical industry, ever anxious to head off any attempts to control drug prices and to gain more rapid FDA approval based on weaker evidence. Gilead, which markets Sovaldi for the treatment of hepatitis C, hired 26 lobbyists to lobby for FDA approval, reversal of the U.S. Preventive Services Task Force's previous recommendation against screening for hepatitis C, and payment by CMS for such screening. (Recall from Chapter 11 the $1,000 per pill and the $84,000 cost for a full course of treatment with Sovaldi.) Half of all health care lobbyists are former government officials.[20]

The Big Picture: A National and International Overview

A sharp increase in prescription drug spending, driven by a new generation of expensive drugs such as Sovaldi, pushed total national health care spending to $3.1 trillion in 2014, the biggest increase since the recession.[21] Based on data from the Organization for Economic Cooperation and Development (OECD) for 2013, the most recent year for which these data are available, the U.S. spent $8,713 per capita on health care, compared to a per capita average of $3,454 for OECD countries.[22] CMS actuaries are projecting an average annual growth of 5.7 percent in health care spending over the next few years. By 2024, U.S. health care spending is expected to account for nearly one-fifth of GDP. [23] Figure 15.1 shows this relentless advance since 1960, together with an interesting comparison with Canada, which enacted its single-payer system in the early 1970s.

FIGURE 15.1

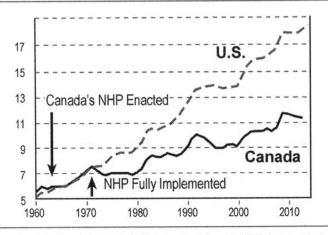

Health Costs as % of GDP
U.S. & Canada, 1960-2014

Source: Statistics Canada, Canadian Institute for Health Info & NCHS/Commerce Dept.

Before this latest jump in U.S. health care spending, some economists and the Obama administration credited the ACA with constraining health care costs. But CMS actuaries are now acknowledging that the recession and higher OOP costs for patients have been playing a larger part than has been recognized. Whatever "slowdown" in post-recession health care spending that did occur is likely to be temporary, and not in patients' best interests. Wendell Potter has this to say about the "skin in the game" approach to insurance:

> *Our marketing folks came up with an almost Orwellian name for this cost-shifting—consumer driven health care. In retrospect, it was a brilliant strategy, and one that got virtually no pushback from lawmakers or regulators. Little by little, year after year—and long before many people outside of Illinois had ever heard of Barack Obama— Americans began putting more of their skin in the health*

care game. They had no choice. The strategy has been so successful that insurers are back in Wall Street's good graces. Their profits keep breaking records, and so does the price of their stock. But what's good for them has been anything but good for a growing number of Americans. Out-of-pocket expenses have gotten so high that nearly half of American families don't have enough money in the bank to pay their deductibles if they get really sick.[23]

A recent plea by two oncologists, sensitized as they are to the increasingly unaffordable costs of cancer drugs, summarizes our current crisis of health care costs in this insightful way:

With ACA now the law of the land, and its retention of the private insurance industry at the center of the health system, the trend toward high-deductible health plans, underinsurance, and cost-shifting to patients will almost certainly worsen. 59 years of private sector solutions have failed. There needs to be a major paradigm shift in our approach to funding health care in the United States.[24]

We will return to that subject in the last chapter, but for now, we need to move to the next chapter to consider how the fractionation of our health care threatens its quality.

References

1. Nichols, LM, Ginsburg, PB, Berenson, RA et al. Are market forces strong enough to deliver efficient health care systems? Confidence is waning. Health Affairs 23 (2): 8-21, 2004.
2. Caper, P. Selling expensive health care lemons. *Bangor Daily News*, March 14, 2013.
3. Berwick, DM. A transatlantic review of the NHS at 60. *British Medical Journal* 337 (7663): 212-214, 2008.
4. Nader, R. In the Public Interest. The crime of overbilling health care. *The Progressive Populist*, October 1, 2014, p. 19.
5. Murawski, J. Blue Cross eligible for $295 million ACA payout, seeks rate increase. *Charlotte Observer*, July 7, 2015.
6. Rabin, RC. Wide variation in hospital charges for blood tests called 'irrational.' Capsules. *Kaiser Health News*, August 15, 2014.
7. Rosenthal, E. As insurers try to limit costs, providers hit patients with more separate fees. *New York Times*, October 25, 2014.
8. Galewitz, P, Stand-alone emergency rooms popping up. *Kaiser Health News,* July 14, 2013.
9. Herman, B. Free-standing ER operator sees stock soar on big Q1. *Modern Healthcare,* April 23, 2015.
10. Waldman, P. For-profit nursing homes lead in overcharging while care suffers. *Bloomberg Business,* December 31, 2012.
11. Walker, J. Price increases drive drug firms' revenue. *Wall Street Journal*, October 6, 2015: A1.
12. Ibid #10
13. Whalen, J. Doctors attack drug prices. *Wall Street Journal*, July 23, 2015: B1.
14. *Associated Press*. Soaring generic drug prices draw Senate scrutiny. November 20, 2014.
15. Japsen, B. How insurers curb costly hips, knees and other medical devices. *Forbes*, October 6, 2014.
16. Dolan, E. Price variation and confidentiality in the market for medical devices. *The Health Care Blog*, February 14, 2012.
17. Wenner, JB, Fisher, ES, Skinner, JS. Geography and the debate over Medicare reform. *Health Affairs Web Exclusive* W-103, February 13, 2002.

18. Brenner, DJ, Hall, EJ. Computed tomography—an increasing source of radiation exposure. *N Engl J Med* 357: 2277-2284, 2007.
19. Andrews, M. Study: 2 million exchange enrollees miss out on cost-sharing assistance. *Kaiser Health News*, August 21, 2015.
20. Demko, P. Healthcare's hired hands: When the stakes rise in Washington, healthcare interests seek well-connected lobbying firms. *Modern Healthcare*, October 6, 2014.
21. Squires, D, Anderson, C. U.S. health care from a global perspective: spending, use of services, prices, and health in 13 countries. *The Commonwealth Fund, October 8, 2015.*
22. Johnson, C. By 2024, health spending will be nearly a fifth of the economy. *The Washington Post*, July 28, 2015
23. Potter, W. The more skin in the game, the more Wall Street likes it. *The Progressive Populist*, April 15, 2015.
24. Drasga, RE, Einhorn, LH. Why oncologists should support single-payer national health insurance. *J Oncology Practice*, January 17, 2014.

Promise: Markets boost quality of health care.

CHAPTER 16

INCREASED FRAGMENTATION AND DECREASING QUALITY OF CARE

As we have seen, the ACA built health care "reform" based on a larger role of the private health insurance industry with a belief that the private marketplace, together with government subsidies, would increase access, contain costs, and improve quality of care. The last three chapters have shown how far short the ACA has fallen in terms of access and cost containment. In this chapter, we will look at two less understood and under-recognized trends, both inter-related and both pre-dating the ACA—the increasing fractionation of U.S. health care and its attendant reduction of quality of care. We will also consider the ineffective results to date of the ACA's initiatives to improve the quality of care.

Increased Fragmentation of Care

Here are some of the ways that health care in this country is being further fractionated, in each case and collectively leading to more dysfunction in our health care system.

1. Shortages in primary care

Health care systems that are successful in assuring universal access to affordable, necessary health care of good quality have one thing in common—a strong primary care base. As an example, about 50 percent of physicians in the U. K. are generalists.

This is so logical, since primary care by definition includes *all* of these basic features:

1. first-contact care
2. longitudinal continuity of care over time
3. comprehensiveness, with capacity to manage majority of health problems, and...
4. coordination of care with other parts of the health care system[1]

Note that specialties which deal with one of the above criteria, such as emergency medicine with first-contact care or ophthalmology with continuity of care over time *for patients with eye problems*, are not doing primary care.

The gravity of the nation's primary care shortage can be appreciated by these numbers. In 2010, only 42 percent of 353 million annual visits for acute care were made to patients' personal physicians, with 28 percent to emergency room physicians, 20 percent to specialists, and 7 percent to hospital outpatient departments, often with considerable difficulty in arranging for follow-up care.[2]

Here in the U.S., if we count family physicians, general internists, and general pediatricians as the true primary care specialties, less than 20 percent of our physician workforce meets the above four primary care criteria. According to the Association of American Medical Colleges (AAMC)'s Center for Workforce Studies, we have an acute shortage of some 45,000 primary care physicians (PCPs) in this decade[3]. A more recent study puts the shortage at 52,000 PCPs by 2025[4].

As the numbers of PCPs shrink, other primary care providers have come on to help meet the demand, including nurse practitioners and physician assistants. Although this has been of substantial help and needs to be expanded in a team approach, they are not a replacement for PCPs' training, breadth of clinical skills, and clinical experience.

Redressing these shortages is a long-term challenge, with little progress so far. Medical school graduates still opt for the non-primary care specialties in great numbers, especially in radiology, anesthesiology, orthopedic surgery, and dermatology ("ROAD", in the vernacular of medical students). Burdened as they are by high debts, often approaching $200,000 or more by graduation, this trend is likely to persist because primary care is so poorly reimbursed compared to other specialties. The primary care shortage is further complicated by increasing burnout and early retirement of PCPs. Medscape's 2015 Lifestyle Report found an increasing burnout rate among PCPs, now fully one-half of family physicians and general internists.[5]

A 2010 report by the Josiah Macy, Jr. Foundation on the current and future roles of primary care made this important observation:

Too often, patients with complex acute or chronic health conditions receive services from multiple health providers in multiple care settings that do not coordinate and communicate with each other. This is especially true for the vulnerable elderly and disabled populations. This lack of coordination and integration leads to a fragmented healthcare system in which patients experience questionable care with more errors, more waste and duplication, and little accountability for quality and cost efficiency.[6]

2. Ping ponging referrals among specialists

With less than one-half of acute care visits going to PCPs, many patients end up going directly to a specialist for a new complaint, who may or may not be able to solve the problem. From there on, ping ponging of referrals among other specialists is so common as to be the norm, all increasing costs and fractionation of care, and all, by the way, adding to the institution's revenues, especially for hospital systems.

3. Changing insurance networks

We have seen some of the adverse impacts on patients of changing insurance networks, such a frequent occurrence in today's health care landscape. Here is what Douglas Holtz-Eakin, economist and former director of the Congressional Budget Office (CBO), has to say about this:

> *The ACA is riddled with wasted money and broken promises . . . Instead of bending the cost curve and raising quality, it has delivered limited access to doctors and the loss of preferred providers. . . . As a result of ACA incentives, individuals may have access to an in-network hospital but not for doctors inside it, or likewise to an in-network doctor but none of the hospitals where he or she operates.*[7]

4. Outpatient to inpatient barriers

PCPs no longer follow their patients into the hospital when hospitalization is required, as was the norm twenty-plus years ago. The management and coordinative role has been turned over to hospitalists, who have no knowledge of the patient or his/her circumstances or preferences. The patient's medical history goes by the wayside except for what history the hospitalist can obtain around the patient's presenting complaint. This is a great loss, often leading to unnecessary testing, ping ponging of referrals, and sometimes loss of whatever advance directives the patient may have wanted.

5. Problems with electronic health records (EHRs)

Based on the assumption that wider adoption of EHRs would improve efficiency and patient safety, reduce diagnostic testing, and save money, the ACA brought new emphasis and funding for further implementation of EHRs. While that assumption might sound reasonable, it has not turned out that way, as these studies make clear:

- A 2012 study found that physicians' access to EHRs did not reduce their ordering of unnecessary tests.[8]
- Another 2012 study found that EHRs raised costs by up-coding of tests performed, and that many hospitals raised their emergency department billings to Medicare.[9]
- Other studies have shown that less than one-half of U.S. hospitals can transmit a patient care document and that only 14 percent of physicians can exchange patient data with outside hospitals or other providers.[10]
- A 2013 report from the RAND Corporation found that many physicians have not taken to the increasingly complex EHRs, and do not find them functional, even after gaining experience with them. This report identified these still largely unresolved problems:
  - Data entry is time consuming, inefficient, difficult to navigate, and interferes with the doctor-patient relationship.
  - Health information exchange and interoperability are inefficient and insufficient.
  - The EHR's meaningful use criteria and the most important elements of patient care do not match.
  - Template-based notes degrade the quality of clinical documentation and care.
  - EHRs require physicians to perform clerical tasks that decrease their clinical care and efficiency.[11]

Decreasing Quality of Care

These following three major problems undermine the quality of U.S. health care. Unfortunately, they are chronic and inter-related.

1. Unnecessary and inappropriate care

Up to one-third of all health care services provided in the U.S. are unnecessary or inappropriate, and some are actually harmful.[12]

145

This situation is exacerbated by the primary care shortage. It is easy to see how physicians in the non-primary care specialties will order more tests and procedures because of lack of information, whether through hospitalists who don't know the patient or ping ponging among the other specialties with EHRs that don't talk to each other. It is also easy to see how profit incentives by physicians and/or their hospital system employers can lead to repeat testing, inappropriate and unnecessary care. It has been well known for years that our largely for-profit market-based system breeds overutilization of health care services.

Past studies have documented that areas of the country with more primary care physicians have less use of intensive services, lower costs, and a *higher* quality of care.[13,14] Conversely, patients in areas with a surplus of non-primary care specialists are more likely to have late-stage colorectal cancer when first diagnosed, as well as worse outcomes.[15]

Patients without a primary care physician seeing multiple other specialists are also vulnerable to being on more prescription drugs than they need, as well as experiencing avoidable drug interactions. We cannot expect an orthopedic surgeon, for example, to have much knowledge of cardiac drugs a patient may be taking. As described by Donald Light, Ph.D. in his excellent 2010 book, *The Risks of Prescription Drugs*, the drug industry pursues a comprehensive strategic plan to maximize sales and profits with insufficient concern for the safety and benefits of its products.[16] And in fact, the industry has succeeded in that effort—although the U.S. is just 5 percent of the world's population, it consumes 75 percent of the world's prescription drugs[17]; nearly one-half of Americans age 65 and older are taking five or more prescription drugs.[18]

2. Overutilization vs. underutilization

The conventional "wisdom" that led to consumer-directed health care has blamed patients for this overutilization, not physicians and other providers who actually order health services. That theory is now discredited by long experience, since increased cost sharing, with patients having more "skin in the game," has not contained health care costs over these many years. Moreover, techniques intended to rein in overutilization, including utilization review and accountable care organizations, have not been effective. A recent article makes this important distinction:

> *Overutilization is a management neologism that has become an economistic health policy fairy tale where costs can be cut, services denied, and hospital days reduced with no harm—financial, physical, or otherwise—to patients, providers, or payers. . . . Real people stand to lose when reducing utilization and increasing efficiency are seen as the primary goal of health policies.*[19]

More health care services are not necessarily better. These examples, among many, make the point. Earlier studies have shown that elective cardiac catheterization, a procedure with some risk of mortality, is overused[20], while angioplasty and stent placement are also overdone.[21] Despite the lack of evidence of benefit or approval by the FDA or the American College of Radiology, more than 30 million full-body CT scans are performed every year for screening purposes, leading to potentially harmful radiation exposure.[22] Another recent study of overly aggressive treatment of the earliest stage of breast cancer—ductal carcinoma in situ (with lumpectomy as the indicated treatment)—found that radiation added to lumpectomy or mastectomy, did not increase survival rates.[23]

In terms of quality of care, *underutilization* is a major problem for patients, who frequently forgo necessary care because of financial or other barriers. These two markers illustrate this problem:

- 31.7 million Americans are considered underinsured because they spend so much of their household income on medical bills.[24]
- Almost thirty percent of privately insured, working age Americans with deductibles of at least five percent of their annual income had a medical problem, but didn't go to a doctor because of costs, according to a 2014 report from the Commonwealth Fund.[25]

3. Worse outcomes by private, for-profit industries

We have known for years that investor-owned care, across different parts of the medical-industrial complex, has worse patient outcomes compared to not-for-profit care. Table 16.1 shows such results for five such industries as referenced in my 2004 book, *The Corporate Transformation of Health Care: Can the Public Interest Still Be Served?*[26]

Since then, we have seen continued growth of for-profits, which now operate 96 percent of the nation's outpatient surgery centers, 85 percent of kidney dialysis clinics, 84 percent of home health care agencies, and almost one-half of hospices.[27] Here are some updates for three industries that show, not surprisingly, that the pattern of worse care in for-profit facilities and agencies continues:

- *Nursing homes*

Extendicare operates 146 skilled nursing facilities in 11 states, and also owns Progressive Step Corp., a rehabilitation provider. It recently paid $38 million to settle allegations that it provided "worthless" care in 33 of its facilities, the largest penalty yet levied by the Justice Department against a nursing home operator for poor quality of care.[28]

- *Dialysis centers*

Mortality rates for the nation's two largest for-profit dialysis chains are 19 to 24 percent higher than for not-for-profit chains[29]; patients at for-profit dialysis centers are also 20 percent less likely

TABLE 16.1

INVESTOR-OWNED CARE: COMPARATIVE EXAMPLES VS. NOT-FOR-PROFIT CARE

Hospitals	Costs 3 -13% higher, with higher overhead, fewer nurses and death rates 6% to 7% higher.
HMOs	Higher overhead (25% to 35% for some of the largest HMOs), worse scores on 14 of 14 quality indicators reported to the National Committee for Quality Assurance.
Dialysis Centers	Death rates 30% higher, with 20% less use of transplants.
Nursing Homes	Lower staffing levels and worse quality of care; 30% committed violations which caused death or life-threatening harm to patients.
Mental Health Centers	Medicare expelled 80 programs after investigations and found that 91% of claims were fraudulent; for-profit behavioral health imposes restrictive barriers and limits to care (eg, premature discharge from hospitals without adequate outpatient care).

Source: Geyman, J.P., *The Corporate Transformation of Health Care: Can the Public Interest Still be Served?* New York, *Springer Publishing Company*, 2004, p.228.

to be informed about kidney transplant options and 53 percent less likely to be put on a waiting list for a transplant.[30]

• *Hospices*

For-profit hospices offer fewer services and provide worse quality of care compared to their not-for-profit counterparts.[31]

Has the ACA Helped to Improve the Quality of Care?

The ACA did include various provisions intended to improve the quality of care, including pay-for-performance (P4P) "report cards" for physicians, wider adoption of EHRs, accountable care organizations, a Hospital Value-Based Purchasing Program, the Medicare Physician Quality Reporting System, and the Hospital Readmissions Reduction Program. These initiatives remain un-tested, unproven, and so far have not been effective in improving quality.

A majority of physicians believe that quality measures are neither accurate nor useful and fail to account for socio-economic factors. Safety net providers and hospitals caring for poorer and disadvantaged populations are vulnerable to adverse impacts of P4P programs.[32] A recent national survey of primary care providers by the Commonwealth Fund and the Kaiser Family Foundation found largely negative reactions to financial incentives and quality measures being used.[33]

Accountable care organizations (ACOs) continue as a high-profile Medicare experiment intended to be "more efficient and save the government money." But so far, it has been more than disappointing, with almost one-half of ACOs costing the government more than expected. Jeff Goldsmith, Ph.D., president of Health Futures, a consulting firm and associate professor of public health sciences at the University of Virginia, points out these basic flaws in the ACO concept: patients do not actively opt to participate in the ACOs, do not share in any possible savings, and hence lack financial incentives to keep costs down, while ACOs have limited leverage to control the costs incurred by highly paid specialists.[34]

The Hospital Readmissions Reduction Program gives us insight into how these initiatives are gamed, rendering improved quality unattainable. It was created with the idea that hospitals should stabilize hospitalized Medicare patients sufficiently that hospital re-admissions in the next 30 days could be decreased; if re-admissions are above a number set by CMS, hospitals would be fined. But here's how this works in practice. Many hospitals are exempted from this provision,[35] while many others avoid penalties by increasing their use of "observation stays" not counting as readmissions or treating returning patients in emergency rooms. This, of course, is just one more kind of gaming ACA policies, including expanded use of up-coding, discussed earlier, to make patients look sicker than they are in order to maximize reimbursements. As Drs. David Himmelstein and Steffie Woolhandler, professors at City University of New York's School of Public Health and cofounders of Physicians for a National Health Program, aptly point out:

> *Adopting unproven everywhere P4P strategies that have been proven nowhere risks quality failure on a monumental scale. It pressures hospitals to cheat, saps doctors' and nurses' intrinsic motivation to do good work even when no one is looking , and corrupts the data vital for quality improvement. As the graffiti artist once said: 'Become good at cheating and you never need to become good at anything else.*[36]

Summary

Boiling the above down, as fragmentation of U.S. health care increases, quality of care suffers. Profiteering and waste has become the norm in a free-wheeling health care marketplace that does not boost the quality of care. Because of continuing barriers to care, including high costs and underinsurance, patients and their families are at the mercy of a largely privatized system pursuing its own self-interest. There is no evidence yet that attempted initiatives of the ACA to rein in these problems, such as accountable care organizations or new quality metrics, will make a significant difference.

Then there's the matter of increased bureaucracy and fraud, which we will examine in the next chapter.

References:

1. Starfield, B. Is primary care essential? *The Lancet* 344 (8930): 1129-1133, 1994.
2. Pitts, SR, Carrier, ER, Rich, EC et al. Where Americans get acute care: Increasingly, it's not at their doctor's office. *Health Affairs* 29 (5): 1620-1628, 2010.
3. AAMC. Physician shortage to worsen without increases in residency training. Washington, D.C. Association of American Medical Colleges.
4. Peterson, SM, Liaw, WR, Phillips, RL et al. Projecting U.S. primary care physician workforce needs: 2010-2025. *Ann Fam Med* 10 (6): 503-509, 2012.
5. Peckham, C. Physician burnout just keeps getting worse. *Medscape Multispecialty*, January 26, 2015.
6. Mitchener, JL, Berkowitz, B, Aguilar-Gaaxiola, S et al. Designing new models of care for diverse communities: Why new modes of care delivery are needed. In Cronenwett, L, Dzau, V, Culliton, B, Russell, S (eds) *Who Will Provide Primary Care and How Will They Be Trained?* Proceedings of a Conference sponsored by the Josiah Macy, Jr. Foundation, Durham, NC, 2010, pp. 84-85.
7. Holtz-Eakin, D. The Affordable Care Act after Five Years: Wasted Money and Broken Promises. Testimony before the Senate Finance Committee, March 19, 2015.
8. McCormick, D, Bor, DH, Woolhandler, S et al. Giving office-based physicians electronic access to patients' prior imaging and lab results did not deter ordering of tests. *Health Affairs* 31 (3): 488-495, 2012.
9. Abelson, R, Creswell, J, Palmer, G. Medicare bills rise as records turn electronic. *New York Times*, September 21, 2012.
10. Creswell, J. Doctors hit snag in the rush to connect. *New York Times,* September 30, 2014.
11. Friedberg, MW, Chen, PG, Van Busum, KR et al. RAND Health Research Report. *Factors Affecting Physician Professional Satisfacion and Their Implications for Patient Care, Health Systems, and Health Policy.* Santa Monica, CA: RAND Corporation, 2013. http://www.rand.org/content/dam/rand/pubs/research_reports/RR400/RR439/RAND_pdf.
12. Wenner, JB, Fisher, ES, Skinner, JS. Geography and the debate over Medicare reform. *Health Affairs Web Exclusive* W-103, February 13, 2002.
13. Fisher, ES, Welch, HG. Avoiding the unintended consequences of growth in medical care: How might more be worse? *JAMA* 281: 446-453, 1999.

14. Parchman, M, Culter, S. Primary care physicians and avoidable hospitalization. *J Fam Pract* 39: 123-126, 1994.

15. Roetzheim RG, Pal, N, Gonzalez, EC et al. The effects of physician supply on the early detection of colorectal cancer. *J Fam Pract* 48 (11): 850-858, 1999.

16. Light, DW. The Risks of Prescription Drugs. New York. *Columbia University Press*, 2010.

17. National Institute on Drug Abuse. National Institutes of Health; U.S. Department of Health and Human Services. Washington, D.C., January 2014. http://unodc.org/documents/data-and-analysis/WDR2011

18. Thompson, D. Prescription drug use continues to climb in U.S. *WebMD News from Health Day*, May 14, 2014.

19. Levine, D, Mulligan, J. Overutilization, overutilized. *J Health Politics, Policy and Law*, April 2015.

20. Patel, MR, Peterson, ED, Dai, MS et al. Low diagnostic yield of elective coronary angiography. *N Engl J Med* 362: 862-895, 2010

21. Wolfe, SM. Many patients undergo unnecessary invasive cardiac procedures. *Health Letter* 27 (4): 2-3, 2011.

22. Brenner, DJ, Hall, EJ. Computed tomography—an increasing source of radiation exposure. *N Engl J Med* 357: 2277-2284, 2007.

23. Johnson, C, Cha, AE. Study raises doubts about early-stage breast cancer. *The Washington Post*, August 20, 2015.

24. Ibid # 19

25. Ungar L, O'Donnell, J. Dillema over deductibles: costs crippling middle class. *USA Today*, January 1, 2015.

26. Geyman, JP. *The Corporate Transformation of Health Care: Can the Public Interest Still Be Served?*. New York. Springer Publishing Company, 2004, p. 228.

27. Waldman, P. For-profit nursing homes lead in overcharging while care suffers. *Bloomberg Business*, December 31, 2012.

28. Thomas, K. Chain to pay $ 38 million over claims of poor care. *New York Times*, October 10, 2014.

29. Zhang, Y, Cotter, DJ, Thamer, M. The effect of dialysis claims on mortality among patients receiving dialysis. *Health Services Research* 46 (3): 747-767, 2011.

30. News release. Johns Hopkins Medicine, December 12, 2011. http://www.hopkinsmedicine.org/se/util/display_mod.cfm?M...

31. Perry, J, Stone, R. In the business of dying: Questioning the commercialization of hospice. *J Law, Medicine and Ethics*, May 18, 2011.

32. Health Policy Brief. Public reporting on quality and costs. *Health Affairs*, March 8, 2012.

33. Ryan, J, Doty, MM, Hamel, L et al. Primary care providers' views of recent trends in health care delivery and payment. *The Commonwealth Fund and the Kaiser Family Foundation*, August 5, 2015.

34. Rau, J. Half of nation's hospitals fail again to escape Medicare's readmission penalties. *Kaiser Health News*, August 3, 2015.
35. Himmelstein, DU, Woolhandler, S. Quality improvement: 'Become good at cheating and you never need to become good at anything else.' *Health Affairs Blog*, August 27, 2015.

Myth: The private sector is more efficient and less bureau-cratic than government programs.

CHAPTER 17

INCREASED BUREAUCRACY AND CORPORATE FRAUD

There continues to be a widespread myth in this country that the private sector is somehow more efficient and less bureaucratic than the public sector. Based on the ongoing mantra by conservatives and their political allies, this has become a meme. But as we will see, that certainly does not apply to the medical-industrial complex. Here we will look at (1) the continuing growth of bureaucracy in health care, spurred on by the ACA's dependence on a growing private sector, and (2) the ongoing challenge of corporatized health care fraud.

The Growing Health Care Bureaucracy

The U.S. health care system is the most expensive and bureaucratic system in the world. As it has transitioned from a more physician-centered to a corporate-controlled system over the last 40 years, there has been an exponential growth of administrators and managers, dwarfing the numbers of physicians, as shown in Figure 17.1.[1]

The growth of managed care in the late 1980s and 1990s was a major stimulus to oversized administrative bureaucracies as HMOs were being marketed by new investor-owned for-profit companies. An ever-larger administrative bureaucracy was involved in setting limits on referrals and hospitalizations, false advertising[2], under-treatment and denial of services[3], disenrollment of sick enrollees[4], gag rules on physicians[5], and hiding perfor-

FIGURE 17.1

Growth of Physicians and Administrators 1970-2014

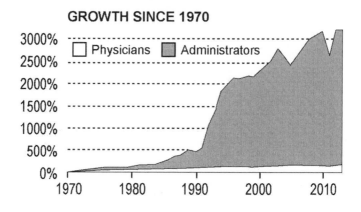

Source: Woolhandler, S, Himmelstein, DU. The National Health Program Slide-Show Guide, *Center for National Health Program Studies*, Cambridge, MA, 2014.

mance data[6]. By 1997, more than 1,000 bills had been introduced in state legislatures across the country in an effort to counter abuses of the managed care industry.[7]

Since 2000, these markers illustrate the growing administrative bureaucracy of the private health insurance industry:

- Between 2000 and 2005, while the insurance market declined by one percent, its workforce grew by one-third.[8]
- Although touted by its supporters as a model for health care "reform" as a forerunner of the ACA, the 2006 Romney health care plan in Massachusetts led to an 18.4 percent increase in health care administrative jobs in its first three years, compared to a national average of 8 percent.[9]
- A 2003 study comparing the numbers of administrative employees per 10,000 enrollees of U.S. private insurers with a similar number in two Canadian provinces, with their single-payer system, found the striking differences shown in Figure 17.2.[10]

FIGURE 17.2

NUMBER OF ADMINISTRATIVE EMPLOYEES per 10,000 ENROLEES, FIVE U.S. HEALTH INSURANCE COMPANIES and TWO PROVINCIAL HEALTH INSURANCE PLANS

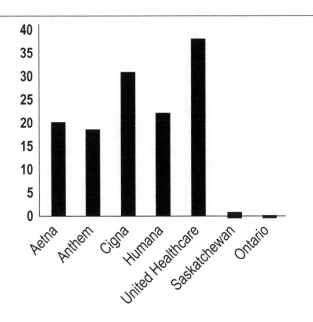

Source: Woolhandler, S, Campbell, T, Himmelstein, DU. Costs of health care adminis-tration in the United States and Canada. *N Engl J Med* 349: 768-775, 2003.

- U.S. physicians and nurses are consumed by large amounts of time in dealing with differences among insurers in drug formularies and seeking prior authorization for planned tests or consultations;

Table 17.1 on the next page compares these time commit-ments with their counterparts in Canada.[11]

The ACA has not improved any of this, Instead the enormous administrative bureaucracy in health care is getting even worse, as these markers show:

TABLE 17.1

MEAN HOURS PER PHYSICIAN PER WEEK SPENT ON INTERACTIONS WITH PAYERS IN CANADA AND THE UNITED STATES

PERSONNEL	CLAIMS BILLING	PRIOR AUTHORIZATIONS
Canada		
Physicians	1.2	—
Nurses	1.2	—
Clerical Staff	15.9	—
Senior Administrators (hrs/year)	23.5	—
United States		
Physicians	0.9	1.0
Nurses	3.8	13.1
Clerical Staff	45.5	6.3
Senior Administrators (hrs/year)	173.7	.03

Source: Morra, D, Nicholson, S, Levinson, W, Gans, DN, Hammons, T et al. U.S. physician practices versus Canadians: spending nearly four times as much money interacting with payers. *Health Affairs* 30 (8): 1443-50, 2011.

- Hospital administrative costs in the U.S. are far greater than eight other countries—25.3 percent of total hospital expenditures—compared to about 12 percent in Scotland and Canada, both single-payer countries.[12]
- There are immense administrative challenges for what the exchanges have to do in determining eligibility for qualified health plans and subsidies/tax credits, especially in verifying annual household income and family size, which are subject to change from year to year.[13]
- The ACA's attempts to set limits on private insurers' overhead by mandating "medical loss ratios" of at least 80 percent in the individual and small group markets and 85 percent in the large group market, thereby requiring them to limit their overhead to 20 or 15 percent, respectively (The medical loss ratio is the insurers' term for their *losses* when they pay for patient care!). But this new requirement has *made no difference* after three years.[14]

- According to recent CMS projections, $2.757 trillion will be spent for private health insurance overhead and administration of government health programs (mostly Medicare and Medicaid) between 2014 and 2022. That includes $273.6 billion in *new* administrative costs attributable to the ACA's expanded Medicaid program, which will take up 22.5 percent of the federal government's total expenditures for the program, more than 11 times the administrative overhead of traditional Medicare![15]

A Continuing Epidemic of Health Care Fraud

Though under the radar for most of us, health care fraud has long been a problem in this country. Malcolm Sparrow, Professor of the Practice of Public Management at Harvard's John F. Kennedy School of Government, is arguably the leading expert on detection and control of fraud. He is eminently qualified for this role, with some ten years' experience as a detective with the British police service, with an MPA from the Kennedy School, and a Ph.D. in applied mathematics from Kent University at Canterbury. His book *License to Steal: How Fraud Bleeds America's Health Care System*, first published in 1996 and updated in 2000, remains the classic in the field.

These examples of typical health fraud schemes in the late 1990s show the surprising dimensions of fraudulent practices by major players in our system, which most of us are not aware of.

*Medicare contractors (fiscal intermediaries), mostly
Blue Cross/Blue Shield:[16,17]*

- Falsified documents.
- Falsified administrative costs and number of claims processed.
- Payment of private insurance claims with Medicare funds.
- Obstruction of federal audits.
- Concealment of poor performance.

Managed care insurance plans:[18]

- Withholding payments to providers, provider networks, or subcontractors.
- Destruction of claims.
- Embezzlement of capitation funds paid by the state.
- Fraudulent related-party transactions.
- Collusive bid-rigging between plans.
- "Bust-outs" (money received, not paid out to vendors, then entrepreneur files for bankruptcy or disappears).
- Falsification of records.
- Kickbacks to primary care physicians for referring sicker patients to "out-of-network" specialists.
- Denial of treatment.
- Charging exorbitant "administrative fees" while shortchanging patient care.

Columbia/HCA, the largest hospital chain in the country:[19]

- Disguised claims for expenses unrelated to health care.
- Misrepresented operating expenses.
- Misidentified capital costs for projects.
- Banning employees and consultants from disclosing evidence of second set of cost reports.
- False claims for unnecessary services, those not ordered by physicians, or those never received by patients.
- Double billing for some therapies.

Professor Sparrow gives us this overview of the structural features of our health care system that make fraud an attractive business for criminals:

- Fee-for-service reimbursement.
- Private sector involvement.
- Highly automated claims-processing systems.
- Processing accuracy emphasized over verification.
- Post-payment audits focus on medical appropriateness, not truthfulness.[20]

In 2009, Professor Sparrow gave this testimony before the Subcommittee on Crime and Drugs of the Senate Committee on the Judiciary...

The health industry's controls are weakest with respect to outright criminal fraud. By contrast the industry's controls perform reasonably well in managing the grey and more ambiguous issues, such as questions about medical orthodoxy, pricing, and the limits of policy coverage. But criminals, who are intent on stealing as much as they can as fast as possible, and who are prepared to fabricate diagnoses, treatments, even entire medical episodes, have a relatively easy time breaking through all the industry's defenses. The criminals' advantage is that they are willing to lie. And provided they learn to submit their bills correctly, they remain free to lie. The rule for criminals is simple: if you want to steal from Medicare or Medicaid, or any other health care insurance program, learn to bill your lies correctly. Then, for the most part, your claims will be paid in full and on time, without a hiccup, by a computer, and with no human involvement at all.[21]

In response to this increasing problem, the federal government has ramped up its anti-health care fraud efforts by establishing its Health Care Fraud and Abuse Control (HCFAC) Program. Since 2009, the Justice Department has recovered more than $15.2 billion in cases involving health care fraud.[22] The ACA has also required revalidation by CMS of all existing 1.5 million Medicare suppliers and providers under new screening requirements.

These new efforts have already borne fruit. In 2009, HCFAC brought charges against some 2,100 defendants responsible for more than $6.5 billion in bogus Medicare billings, many of which involved scams whereby physicians took kickbacks from distributors to prescribe motorized wheelchairs and scooters for healthy, ambulatory patients.[23] In 2015, in the largest criminal health care fraud takedown in the history of the Department of Justice, 243 people were arrested and charged with stealing $712 million from Medicare. These arrests included physicians, nurses, pharmacy owners, and other health care professionals.[24]

Despite this progress, the following examples show how pervasive and malignant health care fraud remains in this country:

- Medical billing fraud is estimated at about 10 percent of all health care costs, or about $270 billion a year.[25]
- Many insurers have been manipulating a provision of the ACA allowing them to get higher payments for enrollees deemed to be sicker than average;[26] in one instance, more than two dozen Medicare Advantage plans were found to be conducting in-home patient examinations that overstated how much the plans should be paid.[27]
  - A recent study found that 50 U.S. hospitals with the highest charge-to-cost ratios in 2012 marked up their costs by tenfold; 49 were for-profit, 48 were owned by for-profit hospital systems, and 20 operated in Florida.[28]
- Netherlands-based Organon, now owned by Merck, paid $31 million to settle allegations that it underpaid Medicaid rebates in almost every state, paid illegal kickbacks to nursing home pharmacy companies to prescribe two anti-depressants, and promoted its medications for unapproved uses.[29]
- Medical identity theft is on the rise whereby criminals steal personal data from millions of Americans to get health care, prescriptions and medical equipment; victims may be unaware of this until their valid insurance claim is denied, they lose their insurance coverage, or find out that their credit rating has dropped.[30]

Ralph Nader gives us this important insight about the economic and political challenges of health care fraud:

> *All in all, the health care industry is replete with rack-*
> *ets that neither honest practitioners or regulators find*
> *worrisome enough to effectively challenge. The perverse*
> *economic incentives in this industry range from third par-*
> *ty payments to third party procedures. Add paid-off mem-*
> *bers of Congress who starve enforcement budgets and the*
> *enormous profits that come from that tired triad 'waste,*
> *fraud and abuse' and you have a massive problem needing*
> *a massive solution.*[31]

Summary

We as patients and taxpayers are being ripped off by this massive administrative bureaucracy in our increasingly privatized health care system, which provides less value and little account-ability as it pursues profits. Ironically, this also applies to many privatized federal and state programs. Instead of service, the over-riding goal is financial bottom lines, often for private corpora-tions. Investors and CEOs win at our expense as the government contracts out growing parts of its Medicare and Medicaid pro-grams to the private sector.

We are also being ripped off by a growing epidemic of health care fraud that continues to siphon off scarce health care dollars from their intended purpose—the care of patients. It seems obvi-ous that a simplified system of financing health care—a single-payer system—would go a long way in decreasing a bloated health care bureaucracy, reining in prices, and establishing long overdue accountability throughout our system.

Now, having spent the last five chapters on the biggest sys-tem problems, even after five years' experience with the ACA, it is time to move on to Part Three to consider what our major alter-natives are going forward toward real health care reform.

References:

1. Woolhandler, S, Himmelstein, DU. The deteriorating administrative efficiency of the U.S. health care system. *N Engl J Med* 324 (18): 1253-1258, 1991.
2. Hellander, I. Quality of care lower in for-profit HMOs than in non-profits. *PNHP News Release*, July 12, 1999.
3. Court, J, Smith, F. *Making a Killing: HMOs and the Threat to Your Health.* Monroe, ME. *Common Courage Press,* 1999.
4. Morgan, RO et al. The Medicare HMO revolving door—the healthy go in and the sick go out. *N Engl J Med* 337: 169-175, 1997.
5. Brody, H. Gag rules and trade secrets in managed care contracts. *Arch Int Med* 157: 2037-2043, 1997.
6. McCormick, D et al. Relationship between low quality-of-care scores and HMOs' subsequent disclosure of quality-of-care scores. *JAMA* 288: 1484, 2002.
7. Mechanic, D. Managed care as a target of distrust. *JAMA* 277: 1810-1811, 1997.
8. Krugman, P. The world of U.S. health care economics is downright scary. *Seattle Post Intelligencer*, September 26, 2006: B 1.
9. Staiger, DO, Auerbach, DI, Buerhaus, PI. Health care reform and the health care workforce—the Massachusetts experience. *N Engl J Med* 365 (12): e24, September 7, 2011.
10. Woolhandler, S, Campbell, T, Himmelstein, DU. Costs of health care administration in the United States and Canada. *N Engl J Med* 349: 768-775, 2003.
11. Morra, D, Nicholson, S, Levinson, W et al. U.S. physicians' practices versus Canadians: spending nearly four times as much money interacting with payers. *Health Affairs* 30 (8): 1443-1450, 2011.
12. Himmelstein, DU, Mun, M, Bisse. R et al. A comparison of hospital administrative costs in eight nations: U.S. costs exceed all others by far. *Health Affairs*, September 2014.
13. Office of the Inspector General. Not all of the federally facilitated marketplace's internal controls were effective in ensuring that individuals were properly determined eligible for qualified health plans and insurance affordability programs. Department of Health and Human Services. Washington, D.C., August 2015.

14. Day, B, Himmelstein, DU, Broder, M et al. The Affordable Care Act and medical loss ratios: no impact in first three years. *Intl J Health Services* 45 (1): 127-131, 2015.
15. Himmelstein, DU, Woolhandler, S. The post-launch problem: The Affordable Care Act's persistently high administrative costs. *Health Affairs Blog*, May 27, 2015.
16. Hallam, K, Taylor, M. Fraud fighters gain muscle. *Modern Healthcare*, August 16, 1999.
17. General Accounting Office. Medicare Improprieties by Contractors Compromised Medicare Program Integrity. GAO/OSI-99-7, July 14, 1999.
18. Sparrow, MK. *License to Steal: How Fraud Bleeds America's Health Care System*. Boulder, CO. Westview Press, 2000, 106-108.
19. Ibid # 18, 7-12.
20. Sparrow, MK. Fraud in the U.S. healthcare system: exposing the vulnerabilities of automated payments systems. *Social Research* 75 (4): 1151-1180, 2008.
21. Sparrow, MK. Testimony before Senate Committee on the Judiciary, Subcommittee on Crime and Drugs. *Criminal Prosecution as a Deterrent to Health Care Fraud.* May 20, 2009.
22. Salasky, P. Government's anti-health-care-fraud efforts paying off. *Daily Press*, March 19, 2015.
23. Insurance Fraud News. New healthcare scams spreading across the U.S., AARP says. *Coalition Against Health Care Fraud*, June 3, 2015.
24. Graham, DA. The true case of Medicare fraud. *The Atlantic*, June 19, 2015.
25. Buchheit, P. Private health care as an act of terrorism. *Common Dreams*, July 20, 2015.
26. Potter, W. Health insurers working the system to pad their profits. *Center for Public Integrity,* August 17, 2015.
27. Schulte, F. Medicare Advantage plans padded charges for home visits, whistleblower says. *Center for Public Integrity*, August 12, 2015.
28. Bai, G, Anderson, GF. Extreme markup: the fifty U.S. hospitals with the highest charge-to-cost ratios. *Health Affairs* 34 (6): 922-928, 2015.
29. Office of the Inspector General. Washington, D.C., October 30, 2014.
30. Armour, S. The doctor bill from identity thieves. *Wall Street Journal*, August 8, 2015.
31. Nader, R. In the public interest. Follow the hospital bills. *The Progressive Populist* 18 (4): 19, March 1, 2012.

PART THREE

WHAT COMES NEXT?
THREE ALTERNATIVES
WITH DIFFERENT FUTURES

Political insiders don't see that the biggest political phenomenon in America today is a revolt against the 'ruling class.'... but the revolt against the ruling class won't end with the 2016 election, which means the ruling class will have to change the way it rules America. Or it won't rule too much longer.

—Robert Reich, professor of public policy at the University
of California Berkeley and chairman of Common Cause[1]

1.   Reich, R. The revolt against the ruling class. *Nation of Change,*
     August 3, 2015.

CHAPTER 18

CONTINUANCE OF THE ACA, WITH IMPROVEMENTS AS NEEDED

Introduction

After more than six years of discussion and debate over the ACA, one might wonder if the political war over U.S. health care is over. We are told by supporters of the ACA that the law is here to stay, and that too many people are being helped to repeal or dismember it at this point. But many conservatives and Republicans in leadership in Congress and state houses are still bent on taking the law apart by whatever means possible. Partisan differences along ideological lines have not changed, and are being amplified by disinformation campaigns in the 2016 election cycle. The war is not over, just entering a new stage in the ongoing conflict.

Unfortunately, this war has been fought over many years with little acknowledgement or guidance from evidence and experience derived from the health policy community. The power, money, and political influence of corporate stakeholders in a largely deregulated marketplace have long dominated election results at both federal and state levels.

As the 2016 election campaigns heat up, with the future of health care in the balance, it is likely that only two alternatives will be discussed by most candidates—what to do with the ACA or replacing it with whatever plans the Republicans can come up with. This would be a mistake. We need to include the third major option—single-payer national health insurance (NHI), expanded and improved Medicare for all, as supported by Bernie Sanders, and assess the advantages and disadvantages of all three alternatives on the basis of evidence and experience.

At this stage of the campaigns, the political spectrum on health care ranges from single-payer NHI with Bernie Sanders on the left, to Hillary Clinton in the center calling for incremental changes to the ACA, to candidates on the right eager to repeal and replace the ACA, rein in Medicaid, reduce spending, and give more power to the states over health care.[1]

As we assess these three basic alternatives, we need to consider two sets of related principles that should be helpful in bringing rational discourse and even consensus about where to go next in our efforts to assure access to affordable, necessary health care for all Americans with the best possible quality and outcomes. Based on these principles, we can then compare the three major alternatives toward still urgently needed health care reform.

Some Guiding Non-Partisan Principles

Most conservatives in other advanced countries around the world have long accepted the concept of health care as a human right. Donald Light, Ph.D., professor of comparative health care at the University of Medicine and Dentistry of New Jersey and co-author of the 1996 book, *Benchmarks for Fairness for Health Care Reform*, has found that conservatives and business interests in every other industrialized country have supported universal access to necessary health care on the basis of these four conservative moral principles—*anti-free-riding, personal integrity, equal opportunity, and just sharing*. He has proposed these 10 guidelines for conservatives to stay true to these principles:

- *Every one is covered, and everyone contributes in proportion to his or her income.*
- *Decisions about all matters are open and publicly debated. Accountability for costs, quality and value of providers, suppliers, and administrators is public.*

- *Contributions do not discriminate by type of illness or ability to pay.*
- *Coverage does not discriminate by type of illness or ability to pay.*
- *Coverage responds first to medical need and suffering.*
- *Nonfinancial barriers by class, language, education and geography are to be minimized.*
- *Providers are paid fairly and equitably, taking into account their local circumstances.*
- *Clinical waste is minimized through public health, self-care, strong primary care, and identification of unnecessary procedures.*
- *Financial waste is minimized through simplified administrative arrangements and strong bargaining for good value.*
- *Choice is maximized in a common playing field where 90-95 percent of payments go toward necessary and efficient health services and only 5-10 percent to administration.*[2]

In its 2004 report, *Insuring America's Health: Principles and Recommendations*, the Institute of Medicine, called for Congress to "adopt universal health coverage by 2010 to avoid needless deaths and substantial monetary costs to society, based on these guiding principles":

- *Health care coverage should be universal*
- *Health care coverage should be continuous*
- *Health care coverage should be affordable to individuals and families*
- *The health insurance strategy should be affordable and sustainable to society, and*
- *Health care coverage should enhance health and well-being by promoting access to high-quality care that is effective, efficient, safe, timely, patient-centered and equitable.*[3]

Based on these principles, which hopefully can be endorsed across party lines if the political debate is held to responsible and civilized standards, we can now consider the first option—continuation, with revisions as needed, of the ACA. The following two chapters will discuss the other two alternatives.

Continuation of the Affordable Care Act

There is no question that the ACA has accomplished some good things for many Americans, including bringing coverage to some 16 million people through the exchanges and expanded Medicaid, dropping the uninsured rate from about 18 percent to 10.4 percent (33 million people), and establishing some limited insurance reforms.

But as supporters of the ACA take a victory lap over the 2015 decision by SCOTUS, they overlook major problems of the law more than five years after its enactment. Far from achieving any of the two sets of non-partisan principles previously outlined, these are some of the inconvenient facts on the ground:

- According to the National Health Interview Survey of the National Center for Health Statistics, there are 29 million uninsured in 2015, down from 36 million in 2014[4]; the CBO projects that we will still have 26 million uninsured in 2020[5], but that projection was based on an estimated 20 million enrollees in 2016, and HHS has just acknowledged that achieving one-half of that number is probably the best that can be done by the end of 2016.[6]
- It will be very difficult to reduce the number uninsured much further under the ACA; the remaining uninsured are a hard core group, many of whom can't afford health insurance even with subsidies; almost 80 percent of the uninsured have less than $1,000 in savings[7]; and there are 3.1 million people in the "coverage gap" in the 20 red states opting out of Medicaid expansion.[8]
- Whatever the number of uninsured over the next few years, we will still have tens of millions underinsured, and will never achieve universal coverage under the ACA.

- A 2014 report from the Commonwealth Fund found that one in three Americans cannot afford necessary care and that the ACA does not address these underlying causes of medical debt: high cost-sharing under many plans, limited protections for out-of-network care, limits on essential health benefit standards, and lack of resources for consumer assistance.[9]
- Despite some new requirements in the ACA, private insurers still have a number of ways to discriminate against the sick, including benefit designs that limit access, restrictive drug formularies, inadequate provider networks, high cost-sharing, and deceptive marketing practices.[10]
- A recent national study shows that 40 percent of physician networks for plans sold on the exchanges include less than 25 percent of physicians in their region; HMO plans typically don't cover any out-of-network providers.[11]
- The administrative overhead of private Medicare Advantage is about five times higher than traditional Medicare.[12]
- There are inadequate price controls in the ACA, which has given insurers, hospitals, and drug companies, and others in the medical-industrial complex new markets with minimal oversight.
- Insurance co-ops were funded under the ACA with the hope that they would increase competition in state insurance markets and give consumers more options; But they have been plagued by lack of support by the Centers for Medicare and Medicaid Services (CMS), low enrollments and net losses, forcing some to close down due to adverse claims experience[13]; co-ops have already failed in 11 states—Arizona, Colorado, Iowa, Kentucky, Louisiana, Nevada, New York, Oregon, South Carolina, Tennessee, and Utah—leaving some 500,000 people scrambling to find health insurance for 2016.[14]
- A recent projection by the Centers for Medicare and Medicaid Services (CMS) estimates that an expanding bureaucracy under the ACA will take up one quarter of federal health care spending and add almost $274 billion in new administrative costs heading into 2022.[15]

Can the ACA Be Improved?

At the political center of the health care debate, Hillary Clinton would make some changes to the ACA, including capping patients' share of the costs of doctor visits and prescription drugs, repealing the tax on high-cost employer-sponsored insurance (the "Cadillac tax"), requiring insurers to cover three "sick visits" a year without charging a deductible, and allowing Medicare to negotiate prices for high-cost drugs and biotech medicines.[16] While she has expressed "serious concern" over the Aetna-Humana and Cigna-Anthem mergers, and feels that the "balance of power is moving too far away from consumers," she gives no indication of giving up on the ACA. [17]

The Urban Institute, a non-partisan organization that studies health care costs, access, quality and coverage, has recently tried to assess how the ACA could be improved. Its basic conclusions are that premium and cost-sharing subsidies are inadequate, that 21 states have not expanded Medicaid, that education, outreach and enrollment assistance still fall short of the need, and that regulatory oversight and enforcement resources are insufficient. It makes various recommendations, all of which require spending more money on the ACA, without acknowledging its basic flaws. As Dr. Don McCanne observes:

> *[These recommendations] are merely proposing patches to the patches. We will still be left with millions without insurance, millions who are underinsured, profound administrative waste, and little means to control our high health care costs.*[18]

We might wonder whether revival of the public option for health insurance could make a difference today. It was conceived as a way to bring needed competition into financing of our health care, and received initial strong verbal support from President Obama. It was part of the original ACA bill as it went through

Congressional committees and debate, where it was killed under fierce opposition by the private health insurance industry and its lobbyists.

With the demise of the public option, co-ops were included under the ACA to address that need, but many soon ran out of money. With the recent closure of the co-op in Utah, the *Salt Lake Tribune* posted this editorial:

> *The original ACA had funds to back the co-ops if—when— they ran out of money. But the Republican-controlled Congress, frustrated by many attempts to repeal Obamacare outright, cut back on the guarantees. . . . Meanwhile, premiums continue to rise and the private insurance sector is consolidating as big firms are bought by bigger ones. There is less and less of the competition that reformers of all ideological stripes were hoping, some with more faith than others, would keep costs down. What Obamacare opponents do not seem to grasp is that, if it doesn't work, if the co-ops fail and the exchanges don't meet the needs of working families, going back to a pre-ACA jungle will not be a workable or ethical option. . . . It'll be single-payer, or at least a robust public option. As it should have been from the beginning.*[19]

But the public option would not have worked then or now. The lack of success of insurance co-ops gives us one example of what would have happened to it had it gone forward with the ACA. Drs. Himmelstein and Woolhandler give us two reasons why the public option, in competition with the large private insurance industry, will never work in this country:

1. *It forgoes at least 84 percent of the administrative savings available through single-payer. The public plan option would do nothing to streamline the administrative tasks (and costs) of hospitals, physicians' offices, and nursing homes, which would still contend with multiple payers, and hence still need the complex cost tracking and bill-*

ing apparatus that drives administrative costs. These unnecessary provider administrative costs account for the vast majority of bureaucratic waste. Hence, even if 95 percent of Americans who are currently privately insured were to join the public plan (and it had overhead costs at current Medicare levels), the savings on insurance overhead would amount to only 16 percent of the roughly $400 billion annually achievable through single-payer—not enough to make reform affordable.

2. *A quarter century of experience with public/private competition in the Medicare program demonstrates that the private plans will not allow a level playing field. Despite strict regulation, private insurers have successfully cherry picked healthier seniors, and have exploited regional health spending differences to their advantage. They have progressively undermined the public plan—which started as the single-payer for seniors and has now become a funding mechanism for HMOs—and a place to dump the unprofitably ill. A public plan option does not lead toward single-payer, but toward the segregation of patients, with profitable ones in private plans and unprofitable ones in the public plan.*[20]

Dr. Samuel Metz, single-payer advocate and anesthesiologist at the Oregon Health and Science University, adds these compelling reasons why the public option is no panacea:

1. *There are few reasons why co-ops and public options should have significantly lower administrative costs than private health insurance companies. . . they still must spend money on marketing and lobbying. Moreover, their per-patient expenditures for care will be higher because private health insurance companies have already taken the healthier clientele.*

2. *No American health insurance plan can survive by selling comprehensive policies at affordable prices to people who will get sick.*[21]

The Future with the ACA

The future of the ACA in the immediate future is unpredictable, depending on the results of the 2016 elections and how the highly polarized political forces play out. But what we do know for sure is that the ACA will not achieve its goals of full access (never to be universal), cost containment, affordable care, and improved quality of care for all Americans. After almost six years with the ACA, earlier chapters have shown how far short of these goals the ACA is. And to boot, we are expending huge amounts of money, at taxpayers' expense, to prop up insurance companies in what has become further private exploitation of the public purse.

The ACA has given the private health insurance industry new life. Table 18.1 shows how the CEOs of six of our largest insurance companies have fared. They and CEOs of other corporate stakeholders in the medical-industrial complex, together with their shareholders, have been racking up big profits while more and more Americans lose out on getting a health care system they need and deserve.

We have only to look at the three insurance giants (Table 13.1 on page 112) to know what the future holds. These giants are already worried that they are not making enough money and are starting to withdraw from less profitable markets in 2016. Wayne Deveydt, chief financial officer for Anthem Inc, sees the need to increase premiums over the next two or three years to realize the profits the insurer (and its shareholders) require. Anthem has decided to sacrifice market share to keep its plans profitable, acknowledging that:

> *When you have fewer national enrollees and you have price points that we don't believe are sustainable, we've just made a conscious decision we're not going to chase it [market share].*[22]

177

TABLE 18.1

HEALTH INSURANCE COMPANY CEOs' TOTAL COMPENSATION IN 2014

CEO	COMPANY	TOTAL COMPENSATION
Stephen Hemsley	UnitedHealthcare	$66.1 million ($254,328 per day)
Michael Neidorff	Centene	$28.1 million ($107,796 per day)
David Cordani	Cigna	$27.2 million ($104,479 per day)
Mark Bertolini	Aetna	$15.0 million ($57,745 per day)
Bruce Broussard	Humana	$13.1 million ($50,319 per day)
Joseph Swedish	Anthem	$8.1 million ($31,016 per day)

Median annual earnings of full-time wage and salary workers in 2014: $41,148

Note: Annual CEO direct compensation includes salary, bonus, non-equity incentive plan, other compensation and actual realized stock option gains and stock award gains. Sources: SEC 14A Schedules, Bureau of Labor Statistics, Current Population Survey.

This prescient 2010 observation by Robert Reich, professor of public policy at the University of California Berkeley and author of *Beyond Outrage: What Has Gone Wrong with Our Economy and Our Democracy, and How to Fix Them*, is where we now find ourselves:

> *From the start, opponents of the public option have wanted to portray it as a big government preying upon the market, and private insurers as the embodiment of the market. But it's just the reverse. Private insurers are exempt from competition. As a result, they are becoming*

ever more powerful. And it's not just their economic power that's worrying. It's also their political power, as we've learned over the last ten months. Economic and political power is a potent combination. Without some mechanism forcing private insurers to compete, we're going to end up with a national healthcare system that's controlled by a handful of very large corporations accountable neither to American voters nor to the market.[23]

As in other parts of our economy bigness is not necessarily best. Neither big banks nor big insurance companies are too big to fail, and why should taxpayers bail them out when they are not serving the public good?

Summary

After almost six years with the ACA, we still have increasing health care costs, less affordable for many millions, increasing pain and worse outcomes for patients, and long-term bankruptcy staring us in the face, whether for many patients and their families, state or federal budgets. We have learned what we should have learned years ago—in the current political and regulatory environment, the private health insurance industry cannot be sufficiently regulated to serve the public interest—it just serves its own self-interest based on its business "ethic."

This is a key nodal point for U.S. health care. Let's see in the next chapter what the Republicans plan to do, if they maintain or increase their political power after the 2016 elections.

References

1. Alonzo-Zaldivar, R. Here they come again: broader health care debate for 2016. *Associated Press*, October 2, 2015.

2. Light, DW. A conservative call for universal access to health care. *Penn 1. Bioethics* 9 (4): 4-6, 2002.

3. *Insuring America's Health: Principle and Recommendations*. Sixth Report of the Institute of Medicine. National Academy of Sciences. Washington, DC, 2004.

4. Smith, JC, Medalia, C. Health insurance coverage in the United States: 2014. U.S. Census Bureau, September 2015.

5. Radofsky, L. Meet the health-law holdouts. *Wall Street Journal*, June 25, 2015: A1.

6. Carey, MA. HHS: remaining uninsured worry about costs of coverage. *Kaiser Health News*, October 15, 2015.

7. Finegold, K, Avery, K, Ghose, B et al. Health insurance marketplace: uninsured populations eligible to enroll for 2016. Department of Health and Human Services, October 15, 2015.

8. Altman, D. Covering the remaining uninsured: not just a red-state issue. *Wall Street Journal*, October 14, 2015.

9. Pollitz, K, Cox, C, Lucia, K et al. Medical debt among people with health insurance. *Kaiser Family Foundation*, January 2014.

10. Patient advocacy groups. Letter to Sylvia Burwell, Secretary of Health and Human Services, July 28, 2014.

11. Andrews, M. Study finds almost half of health law plans offer very limited physician networks. *Kaiser Health News*, June 26, 2015.

12. Healthcare-NOW! *Single-Payer Activist Guide to the Affordable Care Act*. Philadelphia, PA, 2013, p. 22.

13. Pear, R. Insurance co-ops are losing money, federal audit finds. *New York Times*, August 15, 2015.

14. Armour, S. Pressure builds on health co-ops. *Wall Street Journal*, November 5, 2015: A6.

15. Himmelstein, DU, Woolhandler, S. The post-launch problem: the Affordable Care Act's persistently high administrative costs. *Health Affairs Blog*, May 27, 2015.

16. Pear, R. Clinton's health care proposals, focused on cost, go well beyond Obama's. *New York Times*, October 7, 2015: A18.

17. Przybyla, HM. Hillary Clinton takes aim at Aetna-Humana merger. *USA Today*, October 21, 2015.

18. McCanne, D. *Quote of the Day*. Is patching the ACA the best approach for now? August 12, 2015.

19. Editorial. End of Arches points to single-payer. *Salt Lake Tribune*, October 29, 2015.

20. Himmelstein, DU, Woolhandler, S. Public plan option in a market of private plans, March 26, 2009. Physicians for a National Health Program, Chicago, IL. www.pnhp.org

21. Metz S. Personal communication, September 18, 2015.

22. Deveydt, W, as quoted by Tracer, Z. Obamacare premiums climb, but insurers struggle for profit. *Bloomberg Business*, October 30, 2015.

23. Reich, R. Meet your new health insurance overlords. *The Progressive Populist* 16 (1):15, January 1-15, 2010.

The ACA's greatest legacy may finally be the fulfillment of a conservative vision laid out three decades ago, which sought to transform American health care into a market-driven system. The idea was to turn patients into shoppers, who would naturally look for the best deal on care—while shifting much of the cost onto those very consumers.

—Trudy Lieberman, past president of the
Association of Health Care Journalists[1]

CHAPTER 19

THE REPUBLICAN 'PLAN' FOR HEALTH CARE: "EMPOWER THE PATIENT, LET COMPETITION WORK"

With her insightful observation above, Trudy Lieberman reminds us that what we now have in health care is the product of the last 30-plus years of conservative thought in this country. Although enacted during a Democratic administration, the ACA is essentially a conservative bill, originally brought forward by the Heritage Foundation years ago as a way to keep private health insurers alive and ward off national health insurance. The 2006 Romney plan in Massachusetts, after which the ACA is modeled, was also a conservative plan. As Paul Krugman, *New York Times* Op-Ed columnist and Nobel laureate in economics, has noted:

ObamaRomneyCare is a three-legged stool that needs all three legs. If you want to cover preexisting conditions, you must have the mandate; if you want the mandate, you must have subsidies. If you think there's some magic market-based solution that obviates the stuff conservatives don't like while preserving the stuff they like, you're deluding yourself... What this means in practice is that any notion the Republicans will go beyond trying to sabotage the law and come up with an alternative is fantasy.[2]

183

This chapter has three goals: (1) to summarize some of the competing GOP proposals being offered during this election season; (2) to provide reasons why none of them will work; and (3) to briefly discuss the political dilemma Republicans now find themselves in concerning health care.

Competing Republican Proposals for Health Care

The main reaction of Republicans in Congress since passage of the ACA in 2010, has been "repeal and replace" it. Since then, the GOP-led House has voted 56 times to repeal or undermine the ACA, but has not yet come up with any proposals to replace it.[3]

In the spring of 2015, the GOP-dominated House budget proposal did not pass, but its contents suggest where the Republicans would like to go on health care: (1) turning Medicaid into a block-grant program with a 2017 budget cut; (2) repealing the ACA, with elimination of both the Medicaid expansion and subsidies for private coverage; and (3) transforming Medicare into a voucher program.[4]

Following discussions with health care experts and lobbyists, Jonathan Cohn of the *New Republic* distilled these specifics of what Republicans will try to do:

- Repeal the individual mandate.
- Repeal or modify the employer mandate (e.g. change the threshold to a 40-hour week).
- Eliminate "risk corridors."
- Repeal the medical device tax.
- Abolish the Independent Payment Advisory Board (IPAB).
- Introduce a "copper plan" with a 50 percent actuarial value.[5]

GOP presidential candidates have offered a variety of competing ideas, with little substance and no guidance by health policy experience or research. These are examples:

- Jeb Bush would repeal the ACA, eliminate the individual mandate, loosen federal requirements on insurance companies, and shift more authority to the states to regulate insurers; block grants would be provided to the states for health programs for lower-income people, together with tax credits to help people purchase low-cost catastrophic insurance plans.[6]
- Donald Trump would repeal and replace the ACA with "something much better for everybody . . . much better and less expensive for people and the government."; he would put emphasis on insurers selling health plans across state lines; although he was a single-payer advocate in 2000, he seems to have backed away from that now, but his current plan is sketchy at best.[7,8]
- Marco Rubio would deregulate the health insurance market, eliminate the requirement that insurers cover essential benefits, create separate high-risk pools for people with pre-existing conditions, and let insurers charge higher prices for sicker enrollees.[9]

All these are just ideas. The Republicans still have not come up with a replacement plan if they are ever able to repeal the ACA. These ideas just perpetuate their long-held philosophies that free markets can fix health care, that individuals need to be empowered to make their own choices in their health care, that they should have more "skin in the game" to make more prudent decisions, that competition will keep prices and costs at bay, and health savings accounts will allow people to save for the costs of their own care.

There's nothing new in any of this. If the ACA goes away, libertarian theorist Michael Strain, resident scholar at the American Enterprise Institute, defends these ideas in this way:

In a world of scarce resources, a slightly higher mortality rate is an acceptable price to pay for certain goals— including more cash for other programs, such as those that help the poor; less government coercion and more individual liberty; more health-care choice for consumers, allowing them to find plans that better fit their needs; more money for taxpayers to spend themselves; and less federal health spending. This opinion is not immoral. Such choices are inevitable. They are made all the time.[9]

Figure 19.1 illustrates what this means to a growing part of our population.

FIGURE 19.1

'CARE-FREE'?

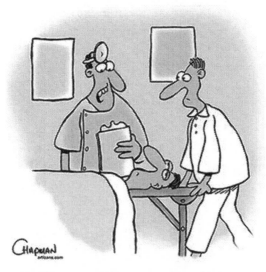

"Hmmm ... no health insurance. Take him to the Intensive I Don't Care Unit."

Source: Reprinted with permission from Len Chapman

Why None of These Republican "Plans" Will Work

These are some of the reasons that the so-called plans being put forward by Republicans are nothing more than failed policies of the last three decades:

- Continued inflation of health care costs over the last 25 years has demonstrated that consumer-directed health care has been ineffective in containing costs, even as cost-sharing with patients increases.
- As the hospital and insurance industries continue to consolidate after enactment of the ACA, prices tend to *increase* as market shares grow.
- If the Republicans have their way, individuals and families might pay less for skimpy insurance products, but would pay much more for necessary health care if they could afford it at all.
- As a result, more people will forgo needed care because they are underinsured and can't afford it, leading to worse outcomes and declining quality of care.[11]
- High-risk pools, tried in many states for years, have been plagued by many problems, including limited benefits, high premiums, extended waiting lists, and inadequate funding.[12]
- Health savings accounts (HSAs) were introduced in 2004, typically tied to high-deductible health plans, with the idea that people could set aside that money tax-free and invest it for future medical expenses; however, very few HSA-holders actually invest this money, and this is unlikely to protect them from the costs of a serious accident or illness.[13,14]
- Selling insurance across state lines is based on the idea that choice could be improved and costs cut by reducing state insurance regulation; if adopted nationally, it would likely lead to insurers shopping among states with the most lax regulations and the least consumer protections.[15]
- Republican policies for health care, if ever adopted, would continue down the track of unsustainability and bankruptcy.

In short, the Republican "plans" for health care defy all logic and disregard experience and evidence of what has happened to their conservative policies over these many years. They are a total disconnect from reality. The Republican mantra remains based on ability to pay, not medical need, and completely disregards the fact that up to one-third of health care services being provided in our market-based system are inappropriate or unnecessary, with some actually harmful.[16]

Concerning the differences between health care and other markets, Republicans still haven't learned from what Nobel Prize-winning economist Kenneth Arrow knew more than 50 years ago—that uncertainty is the root cause of market failure in health care. He was aware that patients have no way of knowing what care they will need, that health professionals deal with uncertainty every day in clinical practice, and that insurers have to confront uncertainty in their rating policies. As Arrow concluded, [a] "laissez-faire solution for medicine is intolerable."[17]

The GOP's Political Dilemma

It may be that Republicans are becoming increasingly gun-shy of their "repeal and replace" strategy for the ACA. On the one hand, their base is enamoured of the prospect of killing Obama'a signature domestic achievement, resents the individual mandate and the intrusive role of government. But the Congressional Budget Office (CBO) estimates that the number of uninsured will increase by 19 million if the ACA is repealed.[18]

That would result in a huge backlash from the electorate, and the Republicans still have no concrete alternative plan of their own. As Larry Levitt, senior vice president of the Kaiser Family Foundation, recently noted about the ACA:

> *It's almost motherhood and apple pie now, that any plan should protect people with preexisting conditions and help people without health insurance to buy it. It's hard for any candidate to walk away from those ideas.*[19]

The latest projections by the non-partisan CBO also estimate repeal of the ACA would add $137 billion to the defecit over the next decade, as well as more in the years to follow.[20]

If one looks at the claims and rationale for these latest GOP proposals, as well as how these ideas have fared over the years, they are obviously false. Beyond that is the plain hypocrisy of wanting to do away with government programs, especially Medicare and Medicaid, from which the private sector reaps huge profits.

Moreover, conflicts of interest through a revolving door between government, industry, and lobbying agencies, do not look good in the light of day. As examples, Marilyn Tavenner, the former Obama administrator in charge of the rollout of the ACA's HealthCare.gov, now heads America's Health Insurance Plans (AHIP), the industry's main lobbying organization; her highest priority is preservation of Medicare Advantage, where private insurers now cover more than 30 percent of the 55 million beneficiaries of Medicare.[21] And as we have seen, private insurers have taken in large overpayments from the government for many years compared to the costs of traditional Medicare. Meanwhile, Andy Slavitt, a former executive at UnitedHealth Group (the nation's largest private health insurer) and the now acting administrator of CMS after Tavenner's departure, sets the rules for his old boss at UnitedHealth Group, which draws 40 percent of its operating revenue from administering Medicare and Medicaid.[22]

Summary

It appears that present directions of the GOP in health care are a bridge to nowhere. Confusion and uncertainty within Republican ranks are also apparent. However, *if* the Grand Old Party could take a broader view of history, re-assess today's needs, and return to the kinds of conservative principles described in the last chapter, they could lead America toward a health care system that our citizens need and deserve. If they do so, they will be embracing traditional American values—efficiency, choice, affordability, value, fiscal responsibility, equity, accountability, integrity, and sustainability.

In the next chapter, we will see how they could do that.

References

1. Lieberman, T. Wrong prescription? The failed promise of the Affordable Care Act. *Harper's Magazine,* July 2015.
2. Krugman, P. Obamacare: the unknown ideal. Op-Ed, *New York Times,* March 31, 2014.
3. Fahrenthold, DA, Johnson, J. Republicans' Obamacare 'repeal and replace' dilemma joins presidential contest. *The Washington Post,* August 18, 2015.
4. Goozner, M. The economic and political consequences of King v. Burwell, *Modern Healthcare,* March 2, 2015.
5. Cohn, J. This is how the new GOP Senate will try to dismantle Obamacare. *New Republic,* November 4, 2014.
6. Pear, R, Flegenheimer, M. Jeb Bush offers health plan that would undo Affordable Care Act. *New York Times,* October 13, 2015.
7. Trump, D. "2016" series on 2015 Iowa Freedom Summit, *PBS News Hour,* June 16, 2015.
8. Roy, A. Donald Trump on Obamacare on '60 minutes': 'Everybody's got to be covered' and 'the government's gonna pay for it.' *Forbes,* September 28, 2015.

9. Chait, J. Scott Walker, Marco Rubio propose 'plans' to replace Obamacare. *New York Magazine*. August 18, 2015.
10. Strain, MR. End Obamacare, and people could die. Op-Ed, *The Washington Post*, January 23, 2015.
11. Brot-Goldberg, ZC, Chandra, A, Handel, BR et al. What does a deductible do? The impact of cost-sharing on health care prices, quantities, and shopping dynamics. NBER Working Paper No. 21632, October 2015. *National Bureau of Economic Research.*
12. Kenen, J. Revisit how high-risk insurance pools are working in your state. *Association of Health Care Journalists*, June 4, 2013.
13. Andrews, M. Few health savings accounts owners choose to invest that money. *Kaiser Health News*, August 28, 2015.
14. Spiegelo, J. Health savers. The consumer finance of health savings accounts. *HelloWallet*, July 2015.
15. Sanger-Katz, M. The problem with selling health insurance nationwide. *New York Times*, September 1, 2015.
16. Wenner, JB, Fisher, ES, Skinner, JS. Geography and the debate over Medicare reform. *Health Affairs Web Exclusive* W-103, February 13, 2002.
17. Arrow, KJ. Uncertainty and the welfare economics of medical care. *American Economic Review* 53: 941-973, 1963.
18. Timiraos, N, Radnofsky, L. Repeal of health law would add to deficit, says CBO. *Wall Street Journal*, June 20-21, 2015: A2.
19. Ibid # 3.
20. Ibid #18.
21. Pear, R. Head of Obama's health care rollout to lobby for insurers. *New York Times*, July 15, 2015.
22. Pollock, R. Obamacare chief nominee pounded on conflicts of interest. *The Daily Caller*, July 12, 2015.

CHAPTER 20

SINGLE-PAYER NATIONAL HEALTH INSURANCE

Promise: A universal health care plan. And that's what I'd like to see. But as you all know, we may not get there immediately. Because first we have to take back the White House. We have to take back the Senate, and we have to take back the House.

—Barack Obama, in a speech to the Illinois AFL-CIO on June 30, 2003

Single-payer has been missing from our national conversation on health care for many years, since it is so threatening to the insurance industry and other corporate stakeholders in our market-based system. The mainstream media, largely owned by corporate giants, want to continue the status quo, which benefits Wall Street so well. As a second-term state senator in Illinois, Obama gave the above verbal support for single-payer national health insurance as far back as 2003. But that support evaporated as early as 2006, when he responded to a question by David Sirota of *The Nation* magazine that he "would not shy away from a debate about single-payer, but is not convinced that it is the best way to achieve universal health care."[1] Both Republicans and Democrats kept single-payer off the table during negotiations over the ACA, with debate over the public option finally dying in 2009 as a small remnant of the idea.

The power of money in politics is a chronic problem. As the ACA was being drafted in 2009, more than 1,750 companies and organizations hired some 4,525 lobbyists—eight for every member of Congress—to influence the legislation. According to the non-partisan Center for Responsive Politics, 2009 was a record year for influence peddling overall with business and advocacy groups spending more than $3.4 billion on lobbyists.[2]

Today, given the failure of incremental reform attempts over many decades, it is long overdue to have a full national debate over the single-payer alternative.

In this last chapter, we have four goals: (1) to describe what single-payer national health insurance (NHI) would look like; (2) to summarize what NHI *is not*; (3) to consider the many arguments for NHI, and compare it with the ACA and Republican plans; and (4) to briefly consider the political feasibility of enacting NHI as an improved and expanded form of Medicare for all.

What Would NHI Look Like?

Single-payer NHI, as soon as enacted, will provide universal access for all Americans to affordable, comprehensive health care wherever they live and regardless of income and health status. Health care costs will be shared across one large risk pool—all 330 million of us. This will be public financing coupled with a private delivery system, wherein care will be based on medical need, not ability to pay. Patients would just present their NHI cards at the point of service, good for anywhere in the country, with no cost sharing or out-of-pocket costs. Today's confusion over changing coverage and eligibility requirements would be a thing of the past. No longer would the first question asked when seeking care be—"Do you have insurance, and what is it?'

With NHI in place, patients would have free choice of physician, other health care professional, and hospital without restrictive and ever-changing networks as prevail under the ACA.

Continuity of care, with corresponding improvement in quality of care, would improve over today's increasingly fractionated care. Clinical decision-making would be between the physician and the patient, without the need for pre-authorization or other intrusions of today's changing restrictions in coverage by insurers.

A comprehensive set of benefits would be covered by NHI, including all physician and hospital care, outpatient care, dental services, vision services, rehabilitation, long-term care, home care, mental health care, and prescription drugs. Bureaucracy would be reduced sharply, with administrative simplification, as with traditional Medicare today.

Health care would transition towards a not-for-profit system based on service, replacing today's predominant business "ethic" aimed at maximal revenues for hospitals, other facilities, medical groups, drug companies and other services on the supply side. H. R. 676 (the Expanded and Improved Medicare for All Act), the long-standing bill in Congress for NHI, includes funding to absorb the cost of converting investor-owned health care facilities to non-profit status over a 15-year transition period.

Cost controls would include negotiated annual budgets with hospitals and other facilities, negotiated fees with physicians and other providers, and bulk purchasing for prescription drugs, as the Veterans Administration has done for years in getting 40 percent discounts.

How can we do all this without breaking the bank? NHI would be funded by an equitable system of progressive taxation in which 95 percent of taxpayers will pay less than they do now for health insurance, and get far more. In his classic 2013 study, Gerald Friedman, professor of economics at the University of Massachusetts, estimates that NHI would save $592 billion annually by cutting administrative waste of private insurers ($476 billion) and reducing pharmaceutical prices to European levels ($116 billion). Those savings would be enough to cover all 44 million uninsured, at the time of his calculations, and upgrade benefits for all other Americans, even including dental and long-term care. Co-payments and deductibles would be eliminated, while savings would also fund $51 billion in transition costs, such as retraining displaced workers and phasing out investor-owned for-profit delivery systems over a 15-year period.[3]

The payroll tax would become the main health care tax for all Americans with annual incomes below $225,000; that would amount to $1,500 for those with incomes of $50,000, $6,000 for those earning $100,000, and $12,000 for those with incomes of $200,000. Ninety-five percent of Americans would pay less than they do now for insurance premiums, deductibles, co-payments, actual care, and out-of-pocket payments; only 5 percent would pay more under NHI. Table 20.1 outlines a progressive financing plan for NHI under H. R. 676,[4] and Table 20.2 lists its main differences from the ACA. [5]

What NHI Is Not

There has been widespread confusion over the years about what NHI is and is not, much of it fanned and perpetuated by disinformation by opponents. Here are some of the frequent concerns that critics trot out:

1. *Single-payer would be socialism, and we're not that kind of a country.* This argument falls apart when we look at the definition of socialism, which means that hospitals and other facilities would be owned and operated by the government, with health professionals employed by the government. The National Health Service in England is such an example. Ironically, our Veterans Administration meets the definition of a socialized institution, but nobody is calling for it to go away. Moreover, American seniors would revolt if Medicare or Social Security were threatened. NHI would not be socialized medicine. It would involve *not-for-profit financing* of health care, coupled with a *private delivery system*.

TABLE 20.1

A PROGRESSIVE FINANCING PLAN FOR H.R. 676

This plan replaces regressive funding sources and improves and expands comprehensive benefits to all (in billions of dollars).

New progressive revenue sources

• Tobin tax of 0.5% on stock trades and 0.01% per year to maturity on transactions in bond, swaps, and trades.	442
• 6% surtax on household incomes over $225,000	279
• 6% tax on property income from capital gains, dividends, interest, or profits	310
• 6% payroll tax on top 60% with incomes over $53,000	346
• 3% payroll tax on bottom 40% with incomes under $53.000	27
Total new progressive sources	1,404
• Tax expenditure savings	260
• Federal Medicare, Medical, and other health spending, and 20% of current out-of-pocket spending (maintained from current system)	1.454
• Total Revenues	3,113
• Savings for deficit reduction	154

Source: Friedman, G. Funding H.R. 676 The Expanded and Improved Medicare For All Act. How We Can Afford a National Single Payer Health Plan. *Physicians for a National Health Plan.* Chicago, IL, July 31, 2013. Available at htpp://0HR%2067 6_Friedman_7.3.1.13.pdf

2. *NHI would be a government takeover of health care.* It would not be such a takeover, just changing to a more effective and fair financing system, with delivery of care left to the private sector. This would be in sharp contrast to the private takeover of health care that has already occurred among private insurers and other entrepreneurial interests, accelerated under the ACA, as described in earlier chapters.

TABLE 20.2

THE ACA VS. SINGLE-PAYER NATIONAL HEALTH INSURANCE

ACA	NHI
At least 31 million uninsured in 2024	Universal coverage when enacted
Employment and Medicaid based, with subsidies for many millions	Covers all ages regardless of work status, gender, etc.
Variable coverage and benefits	Comprehensive & uniform benefits
Multi-tiered system, based on ability to pay	Single standard for all, based on medical need
Limited choice of doctor and hospital	Free choice of doctor and hospital
Fragmented, inefficient risk pools	One big, efficient risk pool
Large Intrusive bureaucracy	Administrative simplicity
For-profit business ethic	Service ethic
No cost containment	Cost containment through negotiated fees, budgets and prices
Unsustainable	Sustainable through progressive taxes; employers and individuals pay less than they do now

Source: Geyman, J.P., *How Obamacare is Unsustainable: Why We Need a Single-Payer Solution For All Americans*, Friday Harbor, WA. *Copernicus Healthcare*, 2015, p.193.

3. NHI will ration health care. This common concern disregards two obvious things about health care—first, that we already ration care under our present system, in such ways as high financial barriers to care, restrictive choices, high prices, and denials of services by private insurers, and second, that *all* health care systems ration care in one way or another. Consider, for example, how the political decisions in 21 states that opted not to expand Medicaid under the ACA rationed health care in those states. Today's rationing is unnecessary, since we already have plenty of money in the system to afford NHI.

4. Won't there be less competition in a NHI system? We have already seen how competition in our present system is *decreasing* all the time as consolidation and oligopoly increases among hospital systems, giant insurers, drug companies and other corporate interests gaining controlling market shares in their respective areas. The environment would change under NHI, when physicians, other health professionals, hospitals and other facilities would compete for patients based on quality of care and service. Drug companies would have to compete based on the efficacy and cost-effectiveness of their drugs, not on the persuasiveness of their advertising and marketing.

5. *Universal health care through a single-payer system is a new and fringe idea.* Actually, the debate over whether health insurance should be a public or private responsibility goes back more than 100 years. Teddy Roosevelt campaigned for national health insurance in 1912 when running as a progressive presidential candidate. It was part of Harry Truman's platform as a presidential candidate in 1948. Since then, although it has had broad public support, it has been shut down by private stakeholders in our market-based system, including the ever-reactionary American Medical Association.

Arguments for NHI

Given the continuing problems of inadequate access to affordable necessary health care in this country, and as costs go up without any containment in sight, the case for NHI becomes more compelling every day.

Economic imperative

The task at hand is to reallocate the enormous amount of money already going to inefficiency, administrative waste, and profits in today's health care system in a way that better meets the needs of our population. There is plenty of money available to fund NHI and still achieve other savings.

Both small and big business would do much better with NHI, paying less for health care than they do now and gaining a healthier work force. Business with international markets would be better able to compete in the global economy with other countries that have one or another from of universal health insurance.

NHI would require a more effective way to make coverage policies based on scientific evidence for efficacy and cost-effectiveness. The ACA postured in this direction by creating the Patient-Centered Outcomes Research Institute (PCORI). But it is banned by the law from making coverage or reimbursement policies, or setting clinical practice guidelines for federal health programs. We need an independent, non-partisan national scientific body, protected from political interference, with the authority to make coverage decisions in the public interest. The goal should be to cover services that make a difference to both individuals and the population at large. These determinations should be based on solid evidence for the efficacy and cost-effectiveness of comparative approaches to preventive care as well as the diagnosis and treatment of disease. Inappropriate, unnecessary and harmful services would not be covered. Since they account for about one-third of all health services being provided today, that would be an additional way to save money and better allocate health care dollars.

Another important part of the economic imperative for NHI is the need to get rid of the huge bureaucracy, inefficiencies, and waste of the private health insurance industry. As Paul Krugman reminds us:

> *One classic example of government doing it better is health insurance. Yes, conservatives agitate for more privatization—in particular, they want to convert Medicare into nothing more than vouchers for the purchase of private insurance—but all the evidence says this would move us in precisely the wrong direction. Medicare and Medicaid are substantially cheaper and more efficient than private insurance; they even involve less bureaucracy.*[6]

Socio/Political Argument

As is described in earlier chapters, growing income inequality among Americans has reached such proportions that essential health care is neither accessible nor affordable for the uninsured or growing ranks of the underinsured. The gap between the 1 percent and the 99 percent of us is striking, reminiscent of the Gilded Age more than 100 years ago. In 2012, the top 10 percent of earners in the U.S. took in more than one-half of the nation's total income,[7] while the richest 400 took in a total of $300 billion in 2013.[8]

This stark income gap has serious consequences for much of the population. Two examples make the point. A recent study of all-cause mortality of middle-aged white non-Hispanic men and women in the U. S. found a striking increase in morbidity and mortality between 1999 and 2013 from drug and alcohol poisonings, suicide, and chronic liver diseases and cirrhosis.[9] Another study of mortality by U.S. zip codes has found that people living in the poorest zip codes have death rates that are almost twice as high as those living in the most affluent zip codes.[10]

In their new book, *Social Insurance: America's Neglected Heritage and Contested Future,* Marmor, Mashaw, and Pakutka have this to say about the political implications of the widening income gap in the U.S.:

> *Social insurance programs engage most of the electorate precisely because they cover common risks and insure most of the population. And because practically everyone is both a contributor and potential beneficiary, the politics of social insurance tends to be "us-us" rather than "us-them" form. Each individual's sense of earned entitlement or deservingness makes reneging on promises in social insurance programs politically costly. Each individual's responsibility to contribute to the common pool makes extravagant promises of "something-for-nothing" future benefits less politically attractive. . . .*

> *Social insurance programs are economically sensible and socially legitimate and thus politically acceptable. . . . Social insurance is part of the essential social glue that holds an individualistic polity together and makes the economic risks of a market economy tolerable.*[11]

Moral Argument

In contrast to almost all other advanced countries around the world, health care as a human right is still controversial in the United States. The dominant culture in our market-based system still treats health care as a commodity, just products for sale on an open market, with access based on ability to pay. When any of us is confronted by a serious illness or accident, with threat to life and/or bankruptcy, we are brought up short in realizing how inhumane, unfair, and cruel our system can be, too often without an adequate safety net.

These words by Dr. Bernard Lown, developer of the cardiac defibrillator and co-recipient of the Nobel Peace Prize in 1985 on behalf of International Physicians for the Prevention of Nuclear War, cut to the heart of the issue:

> *The United States subscribes to a business model that characterizes insurers as commercial entities. Like all businesses, their goal is to make money . . . Under the business model, casual inhumanity is built in and the common good ignored. Excluding the poor, the aged, the disabled, and the ill is sound policy since it maximizes profit. Under the social model, denying coverage to any member of society would refute the fundamental purpose of health insurance.*[12]

Comparison of our three alternatives

In summary, comparing single-payer NHI with the ACA and any of the Republican plans which may emerge, single-payer NHI is the only alternative of these three that can meet the nation's need for further health care reform, as shown in Table 20.3.

TABLE 20.3

COMPARISON OF THREE
REFORM ALTERNATIVES

	ACA	*GOP*	*NHI*
Access	Restricted	Restricted	Unrestricted
Choice	Restricted	Restricted	Unrestricted
Cost containment	No	No	Yes
Quality of care	Unimproved	Unimproved	Improved
Bureaucracy	Increased	Increased	Much reduced
Universal coverage	Never	Never	Immediately
Accountability	Limited	Limited	Yes
Sustainability	No	No	Yes

Is NHI politically feasible?

Beyond the many advantages of NHI, we always come around to the question of political feasibility. Arguably, if we had a true democracy, where votes counted without Citizens United and the overwhelming influence of money in politics, we might have had NHI by now. So where are we now, in the midst of the 2016 elections with their outcomes still unpredictable, on the feasibility question?

On the support side.

There has been broad support for NHI for many years in this country, virtually ignored by the media, as shown by these measures:

- Americans have expressed high levels of support for NHI since the 1940s, when 74 percent of the public favored such a proposal;[13] by many national surveys, a majority of the public supported NHI between 1980 and 2000;[14] a 2009 CBS/ *New York Times* poll found that 59 percent of respondents favored NHI, up from 40 percent in 1979.[15]

- A 2008 national survey of more than 2,200 U.S. physicians in 13 specialties found that 59 percent support NHI.[16]
- Activist positions for single-payer NHI have been taken by a growing number of health care organizations, including the American College of Physicians (the second largest physicians' organization in the country), Physicians for a National Health Program (PNHP), the American Society of Clinical Oncology, the American Psychiatric Association, the American Public Health Association, the American Women's Medical Association, the American Medical Students' Association, and the American Nurses Association.
- Many other organizations across our society support NHI, including Healthcare NOW!, Labor Campaign for Single-Payer Health Care, One Payer States, National Nurses United, Progressive Democrats for America, and many others.
- To no surprise, support for NHI among legislators in Congress depends on the state, with those from states opting out of Medicaid under the ACA opposing NHI. (Figure 20.1)[17]
- A 2013 international survey by the Commonwealth Fund of overall views of health care systems in 11 countries found that 48 percent of respondents believe that our system needs "fundamental changes" and that an additional 27 percent thinks it should be "completely rebuilt."[18]
- According to a June 2015 survey by the Kaiser Family Foundation, 84 percent of respondents support Medicare negotiating discounted prices of prescription drugs.[19]
- After seven years' experience with health care reform in Massachusetts (the Romney plan), the model upon which the ACA was based, 72 percent of respondents prefer NHI to that plan.[20]

Forces opposing NHI

The forces against passage of NHI, of course, are very imposing, including private insurers, Big PhRMA, medical device makers, and other members of the medical-industrial complex. They have successfully warded NHI off over many decades. In

FIGURE 20.1

HEALTHCARE - WHO'S IN AND WHO'S OUT

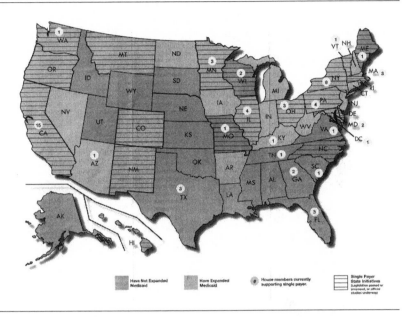

HEALTHCARE—Who's In and Who's Out. Public Citizen. Washington, D.C., 2015. Reprinted with permission.

the post-Citizens United world, they are even more imposing. The private health insurance industry, posturing in its past and present protests about some aspects of the ACA, is finding it a bonanza. The ACAs long-term trajectory, however, is unsustainable. The private health insurance industry would be on life support without the ACA bailout, and by any measure it does not deserve further bailout.

A 2014 Op-Ed by Dave Johnson of Campaign for America's Future, brings us this useful insight into long-term opposition to NHI, as well as other more progressive policy changes:

> *The Koch brothers, other billionaires and corporate groups have been remarkably successful in pushing Congress to pass legislation that helps their interests while hurting the rest of us. . . .[They] put their money into think tanks, communication outlets, publishers, various media, etc. with a long-term plan to change the way people see things. This 'apparatus' has pounded out corporate/conservative propaganda 24/7 for decades.[21]*

There are more than 20 right-wing think tanks that employ full-time "scholars" to oppose NHI and advocate for privatization of health care, further deregulation, and other market-based initiatives. These include the American Enterprise Institute, the Cato Institute, the Galen Institute, the Heartland Institute, the Heritage Foundation, the Manhattan Institute, the National Center for Policy Analysis, the Pacific Research Institute, the National Center for Public Policy Research, and Freedom Works Foundation (founded by Charles Koch). Note the patriotic-sounding names of some that belie their intentions. At the state level, the American Legislative Exchange Council (ALEC), a spin-off of the Heritage Foundation, opposes any single-payer initiatives and lobbies strongly and effectively for private health insurance in state legislatures. Other right-wing organizations, such as the Fraser Institute, the Discovery Institute, and Americans for Prosperity, disseminate "information" that denigrates the Canadian single-payer system.[22]

As so many conservatives and corporate giants in the medical-industrial complex rail against the government, it is beyond irony that they depend so much for their revenues on government health care programs, at both the federal and state levels.

So What Comes Next?

The opening months of the campaigns for president seem to have caught political strategists, insiders, and pundits by surprise. Robert Reich notes that this is readily explained as a revolt against the 'ruling class', which has dominated Washington for more than three decades. Whether on the right or left, there is a level of dissatisfaction and anger not seen for many years. For as Reich observes:

> *What's new is the degree of anger now focused on those who have had power over our economic and political system since the start of the 1980s. Included are presidents and congressional leaders from both parties, along with their retinues of policy advisors, political strategists and spin doctors. Most have remained in Washington even when not in power, as lobbyists, campaign consultants, go-to lawyers, financial bundlers and power brokers. . . . The other half of the ruling class comprises the corporate executives, Wall Street chiefs and multimillionaires who have assisted and enabled these political leaders—and for whom the politicians have provided political favors in return.*[23]

It was no accident that Donald Trump was blowing away the other Republican presidential candidates on the right with his bombastic calls for change, vague and unexplained as they were. And Bernie Sanders on the left was attracting the largest crowds of any candidate, right or left, with his wide-ranging progressive agenda, which is likely to resonate with a large part of the electorate as voters get to know him better.

We can hope for a major change in leadership toward a more progressive populism should this simmering anger come to a boil. These two data points illustrate this growing momentum that suggest that business as usual may soon be overturned in this country.

- According to American National Election Studies, 79 percent of voters in 2012 believed that "government is run by a few big interests looking after themselves", whereas 64 percent of voters in 1964 felt that "government was run for the benefit of all the people."[24]

207

- Gallup polls have shown big changes in the numbers of Americans satisfied or dissatisfied with "opportunities to get ahead by working hard"—in 2001, 76 percent were satisfied, but by 2014, only 54 percent were satisfied and 45 percent dissatisfied.[25]

As the late Howard Zinn, former political science professor at Boston University, social activist, and author of *The People's History of the United States*, has reminded us, "Democracy is not what governments do. It's what people do."[26] We can also draw hope when we recognize that today's times are not what this country is about. As the second president of the U.S. and one of our founding fathers, John Adams gave us this wise guidance more than 200 years ago:

> *Government is instituted for the common good; for the protection, safety, prosperity and happiness of the people; and not for the profit, honor, or private interest of any one man, family, or class of men.*[27]

When we succeed in getting the democracy that we need, single-payer NHI will be a natural fit within a more progressive agenda serving the public good instead of the self-interest of the privileged few.

We can expect a continued and probably virulent debate over the future of our health care as this election season progresses toward November 2016. Most Democrats will fight to protect the ACA as a landmark achievement. Republicans will try to neutralize it, but realize that the President will veto any attempts to repeal it. Their goal will probably be to take the White House in 2016, maintain control of Congress, and dismember or replace the ACA in 2017. The insurance industry, Big PhRMA, and other business interests welcome ongoing expanded markets subsidized by the government. Meanwhile the public is sharply divided over the law, with the latest *Wall Street Journal*/NBC poll showing 50 percent of respondents saying it should have a major overhaul or be eliminated.[28]

Amidst the chaos of our present dysfunctional system, it is high time to seize this opportunity to seriously debate these three alternatives. We need to make a national policy decision based on evidence and experience informed by health policy research, not ideology. This should be a non-partisan process, based on the principles outlined in Chapter 18. If we can assess past failed policies through an honest and rational debate of the issues, both political parties and the country will be winners.

Time will tell whether or not we are up to this challenge.

References:

1. Sirota, D. Mr. Obama goes to Washington. *The Nation*, June 8, 2006.
2. Eaton, J, Pell, MB. Lobbyists swarm capitol to influence health reform. Washington, DC. *The Center for Public Integrity*, February 23, 2010.
3. Friedman, G. Funding *H. R. 676: The Expanded and Improved Medicare for All Act. How We Can Afford a National Single-Payer Health Plan.* Physicians for a National Health Program. Chicago, IL. July 31, 2013. Available at: htpp://www.pnhp.org/sites/default/files/Funding%20HR%20 676_Friedman_final_7.31.13.pdf
4. Ibid #3
5. Geyman, J, *How Obamacare is Unsustainable: Why We Need a Single-Payer Solution For All Americans*, Friday Harbor, WA. *Copernicus Healthcare*, 2015, p.193.
6. Krugman, P. Op-Ed. Where government excels. *New York Times*, April 10, 2015.
7. Lowrey, A. The rich get richer through the recovery. *New York Times*, September 10, 2013.
8. Buchheit, P. Another shocking wealth grab by the rich, in just one year. *Nation of Change*, January 20, 2014.
9. Case, A, Deaton, A. Rising morbidity and mortality in midlife among white non-Hispanic Americans in the 21st century. *Proceedings of the National Academy of Sciences*, November 2, 2015.

10. Wilkenson,, R, Pickett, K. The Spirit Level: Why Greater Equality Makes Societies Stronger. *Bloomsbury Press*, New York, 2010, p. 13.
11. Marmor, TR, Mashaw, JL, Pakutka, J. Social Insurance: America's Neglected Heritage and Contested Future. Los Angeles. *Sage Publications*, 2014, p. 217.
12. Lown, B. Physicians need to fight the business model of medicine. *Hippocrates* 12 (5): 25-28, 1998.
13. Steinmo, S, Watts, J. It's the institutions, stupid! Why comprehensive national health insurance always fails in America. *J Health Politics*, Policy and Law 20: 329, 1995.
14. Geyman, JP. *How Obamacare Is Unsustainable: Why We Need a Single-Payer Solution for All Americans*. Friday Harbor, WA. *Copernicus Healthcare*, 2015, p. 272.
15. *CBS News/New York Times poll,* February 1, 2009.
16. Carroll, AE, Ackermann, RT. Support for national health insurance among U. S. physicians: five years later. *Ann Intern Med* 1481: 566-567, 2008.
17. HEALTHCARE— Who's In and Who's Out. *Public Citizen*. Washington, D.C., 2015.
18. Commonwealth Fund International Health Policy Survey in Eleven Countries. New York, 2013.
19. Gumpert, K. Americans want Medicare to help negotiate down drug prices—poll. *Reuters*, July 17, 2015.
20. Saluja, S, Zallman, L, Nardin, R et al. Support for National Health Insurance seven years into Massachusetts healthcare reform: Views on populations targeted by the reform. *Intl J Health Services*. OnlineFirst—November 3, 2015.
21. Johnson, D. Let's stop searching for a 'messiah' and build a movement. *Nation of Change*, May 25, 2014.
22. Skala, N, Gray, C. Right-wing "think" tanks and health policy. *The National Health Program Reader*. Chicago, IL. Physicians for a National Health Program, 2010: 472-474.
23. Reich, RB. A revolt against the ruling class. *The Progressive Populist*, September 15, 2015.
24. Ibid # 23.
25. Riffkin, R. In U. S., 67 percent dissatisfied with income, wealth distribution. *Gallup Economy*, January 20, 2014.
26. Zinn, H. As quoted by Moyers, B. Howard Zinn interview. *Truthout*, December 14, 2009.
27. Adams, J. As quoted by Hartmann, T. A red privatization story. *The Progressive Populist*, November 15, 2014, p. 11.
28. O'Connor, P. Poll finds backing for gay marriage, health-law split. *Wall Street Journal*, June 25, 2015: A5.

Index

Q

R

S

Y

Z

About the Author

John Geyman, M.D. is professor emeritus of family medicine at the University of Washington School of Medicine in Seattle, where he served as Chairman of the Department of Family Medicine from 1976 to 1990. As a family physician with over 25 years in academic medicine, he also practiced in rural communities for 13 years. He was the founding editor of *The Journal of Family Practice* 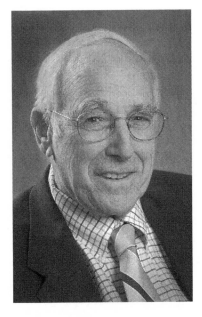 (1973 to 1990) and the editor of *The American Journal of Family Medicine* from 1990 to 2003. Since 1990 he has been involved with research and writing on health policy and health care reform. His most recent book *How Obamacare Is Unsustainable: Why We Need a Single-Payer Solution For All Americans* (2015). Earlier books include *Health Care Wars: How Market Ideology and Corporate Power Are Killing Americans* (2012), *Souls On a Walk: An Enduring Love Story Unbroken by Alzheimer's* (2012), *Breaking Point: How the Primary Care Crisis Threatens the Lives of Americans* (2011), *Hijacked: The Road to Single Payer in the Aftermath of Stolen Health Care Reform (2010)*, *The Cancer Generation: Baby Boomers Facing a Perfect Storm* (2009), *Do Not Resuscitate: Why the Health Insurance Industry Is Dying (2008)*, *The Corrosion of Medicine: Can the Profession Reclaim*

Its Moral Legacy (2008), *and Shredding the Social Contract: The Privatization of Medicare* (2006), and *Health Care in America: Can Our Ailing System Be Healed?* (2002).

Flying is John's avocation, having been a pilot for 56 years. Now, as an active member of the United Flying Octogenarians, he flies patients from San Juan Island to and from the mainland for chemotherapy and radiation therapy. He is a member of the Institute of Medicine, and served as the president of Physicians for a National Health Program from 2005 to 2007, and is a member of the National Academy of Medicine.

Made in the USA
San Bernardino, CA
16 December 2015